REPORT

ON THE

IMPORTANCE AND ECONOMY

OF

Sanitary Measures to Cities:

By JOHN BELL, M.D.,

OF PHILADELPHIA.

NEW YORK:
PUBLISHED BY EDMUND JONES & CO., PRINTERS AND STATIONERS,
No. 26 John Street.
1859.

CONTENTS.

CONTENTS.

REPORT.

This is one of the subjects to which the Committee on the Internal Hygiene of Cities has been specially instructed to direct its attention. It is that on which, in the division of labor, I am required to be the reporter. The materials for the purpose are ample, and it only requires the labor of selection and arrangement to make them available for immediate instruction and guidance in the work of sanitary reform. History, notwithstanding its imperfect notices of the real condition of the people of the different countries whose progress it professes to narrate, furnishes, when read and studied in a proper sense, large contributions More especially is this true with regard to contemporary records, which, while they manifest awakened attention to existing evils, point out at the same time the means of amelioration and improvement. In the use to be made of the knowledge obtainable from so many sources, and to be brought to bear in aid of sanitary reform, it will be safer to incur the charge of iteration rather than of failure to impress the public mind with the vast importance of the questions involved in the discussion, and with the pertinency and force of the facts adduced in elucidation of principles. We must not imagine that a knowledge of sanitary matters, possessed by a small number of intelligent and inquiring minds, is at all indicative either of the knowledge or the zeal of the public at large. Our reform, like every other that has been successful, requires iteration, and again iteration.

Ancient Egyptian Hygiene.—The mere mention of ancient Egypt suggests to the minds of all readers her pyramids and obelisks, with their hieroglyphics, the splendor of Thebes and

Memphis, the superstitious observances of her people in their alleged worship of animals, and of their embalming the dead, both of their own and the brute kind. The annually overflowing and fertilizing Nile, with its innumerable canals for irrigation, is also a theme for admiration. But the wise sanitary measures which secured health to the inhabitants, and their protection from pestilence, by a system of irrigation and methodical distribution of the waters of the great river, and the practice of embalming the dead, under religious sanction, are scarcely deemed to be worthy of notice by the historian; certainly they are not impressed on the minds of the youthful student in such a manner as is called for, both by the importance of the facts themselves, and as suggestive of theduty of a government to exercise unceasing vigilance in all matters that relate to public hygiene. Unless the process of converting the dead bodies, not only of men but of animals also, into mummies, had been in a great measure universal, it would have been difficult to prevent putrefactive exhalations from continually filling and poisoning the air, owing to the difficulty, not to say impossibility, of securing deep and permanent burial for the dead in a land like that of Egypt, the soil of which is undergoing continual changes of surface by the annual overflow and washing of the Nile. With a similarly wise provision of means best calculated to preserve the public health, one, if not more of the ancient kings, made those great artificial excavations, the lakes of Mœris, the effect of which was protection against the impetuous flow of the Nile at its rise, or the too persistent delay of its waters at its fall; and, in either case, to diminish, if not entirely prevent, an exposed marshy surface with its deleterious exhalations.

Carthaginian Hygiene.—We are all familiar with the memorable incidents of the wars growing out of the rivalry between the Romans and the Carthaginians; but few are aware that paving the streets was first practised in Carthage, and that the example was followed by the Romans, or that a copious supply of water for the use of the inhabitants of that city, was brought, after immense labor and expense, by an aqueduct more than fifty miles in length, and of such dimensions that a man could stand erect in it. The cisterns for the reception and distribution of the water through the city were of corresponding magnitude; and even now in rowing along the beach, the mouths of common sewers are frequently discovered. In a like spirit of regard for the public health, the Carthaginians set apart ground for a public cemetery, beyond the suburbs of the city, which became a true Necropolis, a city of the dead, of which notice will be taken when we come to treat of the evils of intramural interments.

Public Hygiene of Ancient Rome.—Favorable as the site of ancient Rome, extending over her seven hills, might at first appear for early habitation and defense, it may be safely said that we should never have heard of the eternal city, never would she have become mistress of the world, if her rulers and people had not early felt the importance of sanitary measures, and carried them out with a persistence and an ability which should serve as models for all succeeding ages. Much of the ground between the hills was little better than a swamp, owing to the trickling down of the small springs from above, and to the frequent overflowing of the Tiber. Unless, therefore, the ground could have been thoroughly drained, it must have remained, in a great measure, uninhabitable; and the seven hills would have continued to be the seat of merely so many separate villages, the abode and refuge of a half-shepherd, half-robber population, who had the Capitoline hill for their citadel; and Rome would have barely acquired the rank of an inferior Latin city, under the rule of her neighbor and subsequent rival Alba Longa.

The Cloacæ.—With not only an intentness to meet existing wants, but with apparently a prescience of the future greatness and dominion of Rome, the work of drainage and sewerage was begun by her kings and continued during the republic on a scale of such magnitude, and in a manner so enduring, as to be unsurpassed and rarely equaled by any subsequent labor of the same kind in other countries. The *Cloaca Maxima* which carried off the waters of the *Velabrum*, at the time a marsh between the Tiber in one direction, and the Capitoline, Palatine, and Aventine hills in another, rivals the largest of the pyramids in solidity and amount of material, and exceeds them all in unquestionable utility. The inner diameter of this river-like trimural sewer was more than thirteen feet, and such as to allow it to receive other large affluxes. "Earthquakes, the pressure of buildings, the neglect of fifteen hundred years, have not," writes Niebuhr, "moved a stone out of its place; and for ten thousand years to come, these vaults will stand uninjured as at this day." The Minor Velabrum was continuous with the marshy districts, known afterwards as the Forum and the Suburra, which were drained by appropriate tunnels opening into the main trunk. In the centre of the Minor Velabrum was a bog or swamp called lake Curtius, which was long an unabated and unmanageable nuisance. The myth of Marcus Curtius sacrificing himself for the good of his country, by plunging, mounted and armed, into this yawning abyss, which was henceforth closed forever, would, if clothed in the language of sober reality, probably read as follows, in the style of an obituary notice: "Marcus Curtius, edile, while superintending day after day, the drainage and filling up of the unsightly and insalubrious Minor Velabrum, and being exposed all the time to the fervid rays of an autumnal sun, contracted a pestilential fever, under which he sank, a martyr to his love for Rome, to whose welfare he gave his life as a sacrifice. Peace to his manes! Eternal honor to his memory."

All these reclaimed marshes became memorable in the history of Rome, as sites for many of her most useful and ornamental buildings and streets. In the Velabrum were constructed the cattle and fish markets, *Forum Boarium* and *Forum Piscatorium*, the temples of Fortune and Vesta, the *Arcus Quadrifrons* and the *Circus Maximus*. The *Forum*, long known by that simple designation, and afterwards called *Forum Romanum*, was a place for public meetings, and also a market-place; it was surrounded by buildings of various descriptions, both useful and ornamental; shops, arcades, columns, triumphal arches, and temples. This is not the time to speak of the historical associations of the Roman Forum, where the Comitia were held, where Cicero harangued, and where the triumphal processions passed. The once remote and marshy suburban village, the Suburra, became after its drainage and the desiccation of the soil, the site of the amphitheatre of Titus Vespasian, more generally known as the Coliseum, and the triumphal arch of Titus.

But, notwithstanding all the pains and expense lavished on the vast subterranean drains (*cloacæ*), it was always a matter of extreme difficulty to keep the ground of the Velabrum and the Suburra sufficiently dry to be healthy; and hence these quarters were the residence of the *plebs* or commonalty. Julius Cæsar, in the early part of his career, occupied an humble house in the Suburra. Of a similar marshy nature was the plain lying between the Tiber and the Pincian, Quirinal, and Capitoline hills, on which a good part of modern Rome has been built. Part of this plain, in an early period of ancient Rome, was cleared of trees, and made a field for gymnastic exercises and feats of mimic war (*Campus Martius*). Large groves were, however, retained, among which Augustus erected the Mausoleum called after him; and behind it beautiful walks were laid out. Another part of the plain was covered with innumerable palaces, wooded gardens, three theatres, an amphitheatre, and magnificent temples, contiguous one to another. To have drained this district, as a necessary preliminary for such various and splendid constructions, must have been a work of considerable labor and time, as we have an opportunity of learning from the experimental observations of an eminent Italian savant (*Brocchi*). He shows that, at any spot over the whole plain, water is readily procured at the depth of a few feet from the surface, and in such quantity as to furnish, were it necessary, an adequate supply to the whole city by means of wells, and without having recourse to the aqueducts. With a knowledge of the buildings which bordered the Campus Martius on three sides, and the still more numerous and imposing ones in the Forum and the Suburra, previously noticed, we see the necessity for completing the simple yet extensive underground constructions in the way of sewers, before a firm foundation could be procured for the more various, massive, lofty, and ornamental edifices erected on the surface. The lesson is a fruitful one, and ought never to be lost sight of in the founding and laying out of new towns. In many of these a proper system of drainage and sewerage is an after-thought, and hence when executed, it is at an immense cost, and often after much sickness, suffering, and mortality among the first inhabitants.

Pestilential Fevers.—Paving, the necessary accompaniment of sewerage, and without which the latter must always be imperfect, was not begun in Rome until an advanced period of the republic, when the practice was said to have been adopted from the example of the Carthaginians. The early deficiency in this respect, and the inadequate supply of water for washing out the sewers, allowed of the extrication and escape of effluvia, which, added to the exhalations from an exposed and wet surface, still in part subjected to overflow of the Tiber, gave rise to those epidemic and aggravated periodical fevers, which under the vague name of plague (*pestis*) ravaged the city and the *Ager Romanus*, now the *Campagna di Roma*, at different times, and carried off large numbers of their inhabitants. The state of war in which the Romans were, with the exception of short intervals, so constantly engaged, must have complicated the features and augmented the violence and fatality of these pestilences. Without professing to have made antiquarian or much historical research, it seems to us that these visitations were not so destructive in the latter years of the republic, and under the first emperors, notwithstanding the greatly increased population of the city, as they had been under the kings and in the first centuries of the republic. The difference in these respects must be traced to the extended system of paving and of sewerage, and the abundant supply of water brought by the aqueducts. Brennus at the head of his victorious Gauls, after having held possession of the city for six or seven months, during which period he laid close siege to the Capitoline hill, on whose summit the surviving citizens had taken their last stand, was finally obliged to retire, owing to the sickness that destroyed so many of his soldiers, much more than to the gold with which it was said he was bought off. The Gauls encamped around the Capitoline hill, in the Forum and the region of the Velabrum, were unavoidably exposed to the causes of fever growing out of this low and unhealthy situation, acted on by the fervid rays of a summer and autumnal sun. Reference has been already made to the ground in this region being sometimes overflowed by the Tiber; and we may now add, that, even as late as the time of Augustus, it was, on such occasions, impossible to pass from the Palatine to the Aventine mount without the aid of a boat, for which each passenger paid a *quadrans*, or about a cent of our money.

The Aqueducts.—On an equally large and magnificent scale with the subterranean conduits and galleries for the purpose of sewerage, were the numerous aqueducts which traversed Rome in all directions. They were nine in number, and conveyed into the city, at distances varying from seven to sixty miles, a supply of water adequate for both public and private uses—cleansing the cloaques, supplying the numerous baths, and naumachiæ, and the houses for all domestic purposes. One of these aqueducts, the Martian, conveyed the waters of three separate streams in as many channels. The first aqueduct, made in the fifth century from the foundation of Rome, was almost entirely subterranean. In such cases, openings to the external air were made at intervals of 241 feet, for the purposes of ventilation. With the growth of the city, and the extension and multiplication of the sewers, it became more than ever an object to keep these underground passages free from obstructions, and hence whether Rome was at war or at peace with the neighboring states, the government, both in the time of the republic and in that of the empire, exercised unceasing vigilance, not only in these important matters, but in every thing that bore relation to the public health. The comprehensive jurisdiction of the ediles indicated the supervision, as well of public buildings—temples, theatres, &c.—as of private edifices, to such an extent that they should neither endanger nor incommode passengers on the streets, but also of baths, aqueducts, common sewers, and control of the markets and houses of public resort—taverns and hotels, as we should call them at the present day. The ediles took care that the health of the people should not suffer by bad provisions, which they threw into the Tiber, nor their morals by bad women, whom they had authority to banish from the city. Officers were also specially appointed to take care of the aqueducts. These *Curatores Aquarum* were invested with considerable authority; being attended, when they went out of the city, by an architect, secretaries, two lictors, three public slaves, &c.

After reading the account given by Strabo of the quantity of water introduced into the city being so great that whole rivers seemed to flow through the streets and sewers, what a contrast is offered to our minds when we turn over the pages of the Parliamentary reports made a few years ago, showing the lamentable deficiency in this respect both in London and many of the great and even small towns of England. To such an extent did this prevail, that hundreds of thousands were deprived not only of an adequate supply for washing their clothes, and for purposes of personal cleanliness, but also for drink itself. The only fountains to which they had access were those of liquid poison; the only edifices to rejoice their eyes, and to which they might claim entrance, by spending the pittance earned by their daily toil, were gin-palaces. In most of our cities on this side of the Atlantic, provision has been made for an abundant supply of water for the use of their inhabitants; and our municipal authorities might, with propriety, repeat the language of Augustus, who, in reply to a popular clamor about the dearness and scarcity of wine, reminded the people of Rome, "that no man could reasonably complain of thirst, since the aqueducts of Agrippa had introduced into the city so many copious streams of pure and salubrious water." There is reason to fear that this appeal in favor of the unsophisticated appetite for water, as contrasted with the acquired relish for alcoholic stimulants, would be received with as little favor in the Christian capitals of Europe and America, as it was in pagan Rome.

Agrippa.—There is no name in Roman history and records so eminent for his numerous and extensive additions to the chief means of promoting the health, as Agrippa, the son-in-law and most trusted counselor of Augustus. He increased the number of the public sewers, and exercised a continual and careful supervision over all of them. So numerous were these subterranean galleries, that the entire city might be said, in the language afterwards used by Pliny, to be suspended over innumerable arches (*urbs pensilis*). Agrippa contrived, in addition to other means, to collect several minor streams into a larger one, and to divert the entire current into the sewers, so as, in a measure, to flush them, as we would say nowadays, and thus to drive before it all refuse and fetid accumulations. He carried his supervision so far as to see in person to the cleaning out of the sewers, for which purpose he used to enter some of them in a boat. The civil authorities of Rome displayed continued watchfulness, in order to prevent the waste of water brought by the aqueducts; and, among other laws to this effect, there was one which prohibited the diverting of the water, that flowed over the *castella* or reservoirs at the termination of the aqueducts, to private purposes, to the detriment of the health of the city, by thus preventing the washing out of the sewers. By the like attention to drainage and cultivation of suburban districts, and indeed of all Latium, the country was rendered in a great measure healthy, and became the favorite retreat of the wealthy Romans during the hot season. These delightful villas could not, even if they were yet entire, be now inhabited, on account of the altered condition of the soil, and its alleged consequent extrication of the pervading and destructive malaria.

Following the construction of the aqueducts, and the introduction of so great a body of water as was conveyed by them into Rome, was that of the *Public Baths*, some of which, as those of Diocletian, were almost small towns, comprising, as they did, every kind of structure for bodily exercise, religious worship, reading, and recreation, in addition to the vast lavacra, and other appliances for bathing in water, vapor, or hot air, as taste or the bodily health might require. Some reference will again be made to these establishments, towards the close of this report.

Barbarism and Civilization.—History tells us of the immense population of ancient Rome at the height of her power, and the villas which overspread the surrounding country; both town and country preserving and maintaining a vigorous and unremitting observance of the laws enacted for the public health. From the same source we learn the melancholy and contrasted picture of Rome, fallen, depopulated, and rendered almost desolate by her barbarian invaders, and the consequent entire neglect of all sanitary legislation. Such was the wide-spread ruin which followed the repeated irruptions of barbarian conquerors and despoilers, Goths, Huns, Vandals, and Lombards, that, in the eighth century, as we read in the pages of the learned and accurate Muratori, a considerable part of Italy was covered with forests and marshes of great extent, and infested with wolves and other wild beasts. The same state of desolation prevailed in other countries of Europe. Rome herself, fallen from her high estate, exhibited the melancholy spectacle of a great city in ruins; the adjacent country a gloomy solitude, and disease reigning supreme over the surviving inhabitants. Plundered first by Alaric, and spared by the ferocious Attila, who had laid waste the whole empire, her greatest sufferings were caused by Totila, who besieged Rome, and cut the aqueducts, in order to facilitate the capture of the city. By this means the country around was overflowed, ponds and quagmires were formed, and the air became in consequence poisoned. The Lombards exceeded, if possible, those who had gone before them in the work of destruction, in which we must include that of drains, dikes, and sewers. Even if these had not been destroyed or closed up by foreign enemies, there were not inhabitants left in sufficient number to keep them entire and to cleanse them. With progressive barbarism and decay of all the useful arts, a knowledge of the very existence, and, consequently, of the direction of most of the sewers, was lost. There was no longer any police, nor the commonest attention to public hygiene. Frequent references were made, in successive centuries of the dark or middle ages, to the stagnant waters in the vicinity of Rome, and their retention in the vaults and the ruined buildings of the city, as a constant cause of taint of the incumbent air. During the twelfth and thirteenth centuries, few of the inhabitants of Rome reached the fortieth year of life, and a very small number survived the sixtieth year. On the advance of the Emperor Frederic Barbarossa on Rome, it was asserted by a writer at the time, that its pestilential air offered a better means than its soldiers, of protection to the city against an enemy. When the Popes returned to Rome, after an absence of seventy years (1306 to 1376) in Avignon, the city only contained thirty thousand inhabitants. This return became the signal for setting about the work of restoration and improvement, and among the measures of this nature most contributive to the public health, was the construction of new and the repairing and opening some of the old sewers. Noticeable evidences of improvement in the sanitary condition of Rome, effected by drainage, were presented in the changes wrought in the quarter of the Vatican, and in that corresponding with the ancient Campus Martius. The first, in the time of Tacitus, was eminently unhealthy, owing to the marshy nature of the ground; but it was so much improved in this particular by the Popes, as to be made the site for the Church of St. Peter and the Palace of the Vatican. In fact, many of the largest churches and finest palaces in modern Rome are so many evidences of conquests over marshy ground, in order to give space and stable foundation for their erection, and also, to render access and occupation easy and safe. Modern Rome, through the Popes, has in part imitated and in part turned to direct account the construction of the ancient aqueducts, so that by means of three of these art-directed rivers, the city is amply supplied with water, not only for the domestic and personal wants of the inhabitants, but for the purposes of cleansing the streets and supplying numerous fountains. The gushing streams and jets sent out from these last, diffuse a grateful coolness through the surrounding air, during the raging and oppressive heats of summer. The most rigid Protestant, in going the rounds of sight-seeing during the dog-days, must feel his *odium theologicum* oozing out at every pore as he approaches the magnificent fountains of *Termini*, of *Trevi*, and of the *Piazza Navone*, formerly the *Circus Agonalis*, or sees a river foaming like a cataract at the *Pauline*.

The calamities which followed the irruption of the German and Scythian nations into the Roman empire, lasted for four centuries; and during this period it were vain to talk of public hygiene. No longer were ediles and questors to be found, nor were similar officers created by the barbarian conquerors. Even after the outlines of a new order of things were visible, and modern history began its records, a long time elapsed before any pains whatever were taken to preserve the health of communities by sanitary regulations. The cultivators of the soil, herding rather than dwelling together round the castle of their lord and tyrant, were badly fed and worse lodged; and both in town and country the purifying aid of the bath ceased to be sought for, and in fact was no longer procurable. The first memorable step towards a better social and political organization of the people who overran and subjugated the Roman empire, was their collection into commercial communities. Ingenuity, enterprise, and taste were rapidly developed; and with the increase of the wealth of the state there ensued greater individual comfort and enjoyments —better means, in fine, of procuring health, and avoiding disease. To huts, and dark and unwholesome habitations, succeeded spacious, if not always well-aired and well-lighted mansions; and avenues obstructed by mud and filth were re-

2

placed by paved streets; while here and there a fountain gave evidence of a recognition of the virtues of running water, and rendered it probable that abundance for use was secured before indulgence in ornament was allowed. This ameliorating process was chiefly observable in the free cities of Germany and Italy; and it was after a much longer period that even the capitals of powerful kingdoms, such as London and Paris, were wanting in most of the essentials for the preservation of the public health. The streets were narrow and unpaved, and with their own mud were mixed up all kinds of garbage and offal; the houses were for the most part small, damp, and badly ventilated; water for both public and private wants, household and personal, was deficient in quantity; and when procured often tainted with impurities. The supply of food was irregular, and never in the variety required for the purposes of health. In all the cities of Europe, in the middle ages, the population was excessive, owing to the insecurity of persons and property outside the walls during their frequent and almost continual wars, and to the consequent flight of large numbers from the country, who sought refuge in the city from the sudden fury of a barbarous enemy. It mattered but little whether the town were large or small; there was always a disproportion between the number of its inhabitants and the space for habitation and change of air Hence we cannot be surprised that any noticeable deviation from the customary states of the atmosphere, or, still more, interruption to the regular supply of food, should have been followed in city, town, and hamlet, with pestilence in its most appalling and deadly forms. Even if we were ignorant of all the particulars of bad medical police, or of its entire neglect, and of the mode of living during this period, we still could not fail to see in these melancholy chapters of the devastations from epidemic diseases, a want of adequate public hygiene, if not a total ignorance of its principles. In proportion, on the other hand, to more conformity with, and a better appreciation of, these latter, was there an abatement, if not entire disappearance of these scourges of mankind. Sanitary measures, methodically carried out, were followed by improved public health and increased duration of the life of the individual.

Vital statistics enable us to speak with confidence of the progressive ameliorations, in these respects, which accompanied advancing civilization. The mortality in Paris in the early part of the fourteenth century has been estimated from a manuscript document to be 1 in 20; whereas the average mortality of the inhabitants of that city, in the very poorest arrondissement or ward, as we might term it, in which poverty and destitution are extreme, was 1 in 24, in the first third of the present century. The average deaths in all Paris at the same date (1830) was 1 in 32, and among the more wealthy inhabitants, 1 in 42; and hence we are safe in saying that the mechanic of the present day, who resides in the French capital, is better off on the score of air and the appliances for supporting life, than the rich inhabitant at the opening of the thirteenth century, notwithstanding that the population is more than 300 times greater now than it was then. The difference in the vital statistics of the two periods thus compared is easily explained by the entire neglect of public hygiene in the former, and the careful attention which it receives in the latter. Although paving of the streets of Paris had been begun in the twelfth century, under Philip Augustus, yet it was of very limited extent at the beginning of the fourteenth, when Philip the Fair was king. At that time the streets of Paris gave out abominable stenches, so obstructed where they with mud, dung, and other excrementitial substances and offal of all kinds. Even towards the close of the century things were no better, if we may judge from a proclamation of Charles VI., which speaks of the pavement being so broken up into ruts, that it was dangerous in many places to ride either on horseback or in a carriage; and that, owing to the accumulation of refuse of all kinds, grave diseases and death were common. With few exceptions, the houses were little better than hovels. Even down to the early period of the reign of Louis XIV., the greater number of the streets were still unpaved, or paved only on one side and at certain distances; they were obstructed also by the same kind of abominations already mentioned. Historians remark that, after the paving of Dijon, the ancient capital of Burgundy, in the middle of the fourteenth century, dysentery, spotted fever, and other diseases became of less frequent occurrence in that city. A still more striking example of the effect of improved sanitary legislation in increasing the average duration of human life, is exhibited in the registration of the births and deaths, and of the population of the city of Geneva, during the last three centuries. M. Marc d'Espine, in a late work on "Comparative Mortuary Statistics," shows, that the *probable* life at Geneva in the sixteenth century was rather less than 5 years; in the seventeenth century 11 years; at the beginning of the eighteenth 27 years; at the end of the century 32 years; and now it is 44 years. M. Mallet had previously ascertained from the same documents, that the mean duration of life in Geneva, in 1833, was nearly the double (or as 40 years 5 months to 21 years 2 months) of that reached rather more than two centuries before.

Causes of Pestilence.—Nearly all the great cities of the world have been founded on the banks and at the confluence of rivers, or on the sea-shore, where the ground is low, flat, and often marshy, and liable to be in part flooded by heavy rains, or the overflow of adjoining rivers. In localities like these, almost invariably at particular seasons, and under certain regularly recurring atmospherical influences, fevers of a periodical kind afflict the first inhabitants. It was so, as we have already stated, at Rome; and in the cities and small towns, too, of modern Europe, as well as those in America, the same unfavorable localities have produced the same effect, until the industry and art of the inhabitants have been exerted to alter the surface of the ground by firm pavements and judicious draining, so that the water coming from the houses, and that falling in the streets in the shape of rain, shall readily flow into the sewers beneath, in place of being allowed to stagnate in ruts, hollows, and pools, and afterwards, with the aid of heat, to bring about a putrefactive fermentation of all the refuse accumulated, in the shape of vegetable and animal offal, and other matters which are thrown or otherwise find their way into the streets. A compost thus formed of all kinds of abominations, in union with the filth retained in most of the houses of Europe during the middle ages, was a perpetually sustaining cause, not only of periodical fevers, but of plague itself. The meterials of wood, and lath, and plaster, of which the houses were chiefly built, by retaining moisture and yielding to decay, must have greatly contributed to the evolution of foul and unwholesome air, which was added to the permanent supply in the streets. Fire in some instances came opportunely to purify the air, while it destroyed the dwellings in a city. The great fire of London in 1665, which followed the great plague, destroyed thirteen thousand houses and eighty-nine churches, in four hundred streets; but it left the English capital free, ever after, from the plague. The benefits would have been much more complete if the streets had been laid out after a general and uniform plan, instead of preserving the old lines, although many of them were made wider. To this last circumstance, and the better construction of the houses, both as regards the material, brick, and the larger access of light and air, was the new city indebted for a higher sanitary standard than it had ever attained before. But the imperfect paving and drainage of London still left it open to intermittent fever and dysentry, both of which prevailed every year. It will surprise many persons, general readers too, when they are told that the mortality from the former cause alone, in a population at the time not greater than that of Philadelphia, was from one to two thousand persons annually. Now, it scarcely figures on the mortuary list, owing to the great sanitary improvements in the metropolis, especially under the heads just mentioned. In former times, it appears that Walbrook, Sherbourne, Longbourne, and Oldbourne, were really brooks, often closed up by filth, and in some places the currents so much obstructed as to form pools. A large portion of the country also, around London, was a marsh, and indeed the banks of the Thames, from Lambeth to Woolwich, was one continued swamp. All these parts, however, have been underdrained, extensive sewers formed, the ditches filled up, the river banked out, and the site generally rendered so dry, that London is now unquestionably not only the most healthy capital in Europe, but on the score of salubrity, is scarcely rivaled by any city in the world.

Venice.—We have been accustomed to read and to speak of the wonderful and almost miraculous progress of Rome, from a small and insignificant beginning to universal empire, and to expatiate on the firmness, courage, and martial spirit of her people, which bore them up under the most trying and adverse circumstances. Viewed under another, and hygienic aspect, her career must excite our surprise and admiration to a still geater extent, when we reflect on the eminently unfavorable geographical situation of the city, as every way adverse to health, and to the growth in numbers, wealth, and splendor which she ultimately attained. It would indeed be difficult to adduce a stronger and more convincing proof of the importance of sanitary measures, not only for the prosperity, but for the existence of a city, than was exhibited in the history of Rome. But in more modern times the same instructive lessons have been taught, with even greater force and point, by the foundation and growth of the three great cities of Venice, Amsterdam, and St. Petersburg. Had the refugees from the mainland, who fled, before Attila and his Huns, to the small islands in the lagunes of the Adriatic, hesitated to procure a stable and permanent abiding-place for themselves amid the waters, and to set about laying at once the foundations of a mart for commerce, they might, perhaps, have had a line in history, telling of their love of freedom and of their success as fishermen and buccaneers, but never would the world have heard of the name of Venice, or of its extensive trade and political power. Never would the spectacle have been exhibited of a great city rising as it were out of the sea, and resplendent with marble palaces, and churches, and piazzas, and with rich tessellated pavements, and houses, many of them, palatial in size and architectural decorations, and nearly all of these edifices, both public and private, built on piers. There was pavement-foundation of a new kind, and upon a large and costly scale; but how fully was the expense repaid! Where canals take, in most cases, the place of streets, these are necessarily small, if not insignificant; but their pavements required a heavier outlay than that of many of the broad avenues of other cities. What shall be said of the engineering skill in making the canals, and in preserving their requisite levels, as well as of the labor in preventing undue accumulations of offal and refuse of all kinds cast into them. The entire exemption of the inhabitants of Venice from periodical fevers, is well calculated to excite surprise under any view which may be taken of the peculiar topographical features of the city. During the summer months the lagunes give out very unpleasant odors.

Amsterdam had as small and unpropitious beginning as the Queen of the Adriatic, and like that of the latter, it was a maritime one. Its founders were, first, a few fishermen, and then a few traders, whose early efforts were directed to prevent them from sinking in the morasses on which they had erected their humble dwellings, and from having these swept away by the sudden rising of the stormy Zuyder Zee. Drainage by canals gave them something like *terra firma* in their marshes, while dykes sheltered them from the capricious fury of the ocean. Industry and enterprise thus early exercised were not long in being directed into the channels of an extensive and lucrative commerce, which brought the inhabitants wealth and a mercantile marine. Its tonnage constituted a large part of that of the Seven United Provinces, and this, at the close of the seventeenth century, was nearly equal to the tonnage of all the rest of Europe. Amsterdam presents the spectacle of a flourishing and handsomely-built city, of more than two hundred thousand inhabitants, with well-paved and clean streets, which sometimes run parallel to, and sometimes are intersected by, numerous canals, and with public and private edifices evincing durability, taste, and wealth. The whole of them rest on piles; and hence the common remark, assuming the tone of complaint, that a house costs as much below as above the ground. It should be remembered, however, that a house is worth little above-ground anywhere, as a residence, unless the under-ground be well kept, and rest on a dry and properly-drained soil. Notwithstanding, however, all the pains taken to keep the canals of Amsterdam clear of accumulations of filth or other obstruction, the depth of water is often insufficient to prevent offensive and injurious exhalations, which affect the health and lessen the mean duration of the life of the inhabitants. What is here said of Amsterdam applies to nearly all Holland. The people of that country, inhabiting a barren soil, alternately marsh and sand, and almost submerged by water, and breathing an atmosphere the most unfriendly to human comfort, so far from retiring before the encroachments of the ocean, erect barriers to restrain its fury, give new channels to their sluggish waves, drain by numerous canals their marshes and morasses, and convert, as it were, the elements which seemed to be the means of destruction, into so many sources of wealth and power.

St. Petersburg, the capital of the Russian empire, rests, like Venice and Amsterdam, on made ground, once an area of marsh and bog, near the mouth of the Neva. Its foundation, unlike, however, that of the free cities just named, was owing to the despotic will of one man, Peter the Great, who triumphed over nature, but at an enormous sacrifice of human life. History tells of forty thousand men having been employed at one time in the preliminary work of draining of the soil, and filling up pools and quagmires; and of three hundred thousand men having lost their lives before the work was completed. Now, we look at a magnificent capital, containing a population of half a million of souls, with its wide and long streets, its grand stone quays extending for three miles on each side of the Neva, its apparently endless lines of imposing houses in a uniform style of architecture for entire blocks and even streets, interspersed with churches and palaces and government edifices. All this has been created within the period that has elapsed since the foundation and first settlement of Philadelphia. Well might it be said, after a study of the rise and growth of all the great capitals and celebrated cities of the world, that the first and the most important chapter in the history of civilization is that of drainage. If there be exceptions, they will be found, for the most part, to strengthen and enforce the general practice, by showing the inconveniences and loss caused by its neglect.

Berlin.—As a part of the contrasted picture of neglect of the most important measures of sanitary legislation in cities, we may adduce the instance of Berlin, the capital of Prussia. For the first half of the seventeenth century, its streets were not entirely paved; and at the beginning of the century they were never swept. The new market was paved as late as 1679. How different the state of things in the commercial and free city of Augsburg, the paving of which was begun in the early part of the fifteenth century; and in the earliest periods it had subterranean passages or sewers. In Berlin, on the other hand, in the latter part of the seventeenth century (1671), every countryman who came to the market was required to carry away with him a load of dirt. Hog-styes were erected on the streets, sometimes under the windows. Berlin had no regular sewers or underground drains at as recent a date as 1846. A sluggish but considerable river, the Spree, almost stagnates in the town. It might be made a grand cloaque, connecting with the other drains when covered, and the whole of them, as well as the streets, could be washed by water raised by engines, at a cost not greater than that now incurred for stucco work, and other outside decorations for the houses. Large puddles of filth are allowed to collect before the doors even of the best houses, which, especially in the last months of summer, diffuse a most horrible stench. It must be admitted, however, that the low situation of the town renders drainage a matter of great difficulty. Laing, the traveler, speaking of Berlin as he found it 1841, says: "It is a fine city, very like the age she represents—very fine, and very nasty. The streets are spacious and straight, with broad margins on each side for foot-passengers; and a band of broad flag-stones on their margins, make them much more walkable than the streets of most continental towns. But these margins are divided from the spacious carriage-way in the middle by open kennels, telling the most unutterable things. These open kennels are boarded over only at the gateways of the palaces, to let the carriages cross them, and must be particularly convenient to the inhabitants, for they are not at all particularly agreeable." "If bronze and marble could smell, Blucher and Bulow, Schwerin and Ziethen, and duck-winged angels, and two-headed eagles innumerable, would be found on their pedestals, holding their noses instead of grasping [as in the case of the generals] their swords." Berlin is still so far behindhand in the comforts of life, as not to have water conveyed in pipes into the city and the houses. "Three hundred thousand people have taste enough to be in dreamy ecstasies at the singing of Madame Pasta, or the dancing of Taglioni, and have not taste enough to appreciate or feel the want of a supply of water in their kitchens, sculleries, drains, sewers, and water-closets." No surprise need be felt that Berlin was scourged with the cholera in 1831, and again with still greater severity in 1837. Putting aside drainage, the Prussian capital is, in the width and general arrangements of the streets, and the better ventilation of the houses, superior to the French; but yet the proportionate mortality from Cholera was much greater, or at the rate of nearly 2½ to 1 in 1831, in the former than in the latter city—which, as commonly described, was so great a sufferer. In the second attack (in 1837), the mortality was still heavier in Berlin, or, as the difference between 1426 and 2174 deaths. There, as in nearly every city in which the Cholera made its attack, the greater number of cases, and the chief mortality, were found in dark, narrow streets, inaccessible to the rays of the sun and to winds, and in low, damp habitations, especially near the water.

Neglect of Sanitary Legislation.—During the last two centuries, colonization and incidental conquest have exerted a powerful influence on the political and social relations of the different countries in both hemispheres, from which neither Hindoo nor Chinese, Turk nor Tartar, Indian nor Negro are exempt. Consequent upon the vast extension and the openings of new channels of commerce, have been the foundation and growth of many cities, the inhabitants of which, in their eagerness for gain, have hardly allowed themselves, until recently, time to attend to the obvious requirements of public hygiene. Looking too much at the surface, they have often neglected proper draining and sewerage, and the means of procuring an adequate supply of water; and, more surprising still, a renewal of fresh air by suitable ventilation. The consequences of this neglect have been the production of febrile and other diseases, which have not only destroyed life to a fearful extent, but retarded industry and greatly interfered with social progress and educational amelioration. These evils are not confined to Calcutta and New Orleans, to Cairo and Constantinople; they are but too apparent in Liverpool and Manchester, and Glasgow, and New York; and, although in less degree, in Boston, Philadelphia, and Baltimore, not to speak of our great inland towns on the Mississippi and its tributaries, and on our great Lakes. Little admonished by the history of former ages, the people of Europe and America have paid but scant attention to the best measures for preventing diseases, and for preserving health among the masses. The poor, and the destitute, and the degraded, have been too long allowed to remain in their ignorance, to grovel in their filth, and while suffering acutely themselves, to spread around them the contamination and contagion of the diseases of body and of mind, which inevitably result from their neglected condition. The philanthropic few have, from time to time, remonstrated: they have also recommended, and as far as their limited efforts would allow, have carried out improvements; but the former have never obtained a full public hearing, and the latter were too partial in their nature to prune, still less to eradicate, the wide-spread and constantly growing evils. The Plague of Asia and Africa, the Yellow Fever of America, the Typhus Fever in Europe, and the Cholera in all quarters of the world, have spread fright and death, have elicited many legislative and municipal enactments, and given rise to acts of heroic devotion for the relief of suffering and humanity; but until a recent period they have failed, notwithstanding their frequent and dreaded visits, to fix the attention of the several communities, among which they have been most rife, on their real, and as far as could be ascertained, their preventible causes. It is under these circumstances that Hygeia may be invoked, not merely as the handmaid of Medicine, but as the potent divinity saving her tens of thousands of lives, while the latter can only hope to rescue her hundreds, after incredible efforts and expense on the part of her immediate votaries.

Concurrently with the increase, and both as an effect, and, in turn, a cause of commerce, have been the vast extension and multiplication of manufactures within the past century, and the concentration of human beings, in consequence, far beyond what would be allowable on any principle of hygiene. Deprived, as so many tens of thousands are, in the great manufacturing cities and towns of Great Britain and France, of the common air and common light, pent up in close and damp, often underground lodgings by night, and forced to extraordinary and yet partial bodily efforts by day, receiving an inadequate supply of food, and tempted by their overpowering feelings of exhaustion and depression to seek for temporary renovation and excitement in the use of ardent spirits, or fermented and drugged, erst called malt liquors, what wonder that they are invaded by disease in every shape—fevers, pulmonary consumption, scrofula, and all that can disfigure and deform? The picture is a gloomy one, and suggestive of fearful forebodings; it has long enlisted the sympathies of the benevolent, and has at last startled the selfish and the avaricious, who feel a well-grounded alarm at the probability of the continued sufferings and degradation of a neglected, if not despised, class of their fellow-beings diminishing their own gains. But we must not scrutinize motives too closely, if the acts be of an ameliorating and kindly nature. Enlightened public spirit is urging those who have the power, to make the requisite reforms, and in legislative enactments, as well as in voluntary associations and individual liberality, satisfactory proofs are given of a new and better state of things. Recurrence will soon be made to this subject. In some of the towns of England, of late years, public baths have been opened, and public wash-houses erected, so as to insure to the poorer classes cleanliness of person and clothing, two great means of preserving health, and, indirectly, of aiding the cause of morals; the mind receiving from the body's purity a secret sympathetic aid.

The burden of sanitary legislation is protection of the public health, compatibly with the rights of person and property, and the pursuits of industry. The common right of all is entire enjoyment of the material conditions for healthy life. This right is seldom obtained in its full latitude. It is too often neglected by those who might, with care, enjoy it; and, still oftener, it is withheld or violated by force or selfishness in such a way that the people in mass find it difficult to obtain justice. The contest between cupidity and sanitary rights is sometimes unavoidable, but more frequently it arises from the ignorance on the part of the opponents of reform. So soon as people are congregated in cities and other marts of business, they discover, on coming to a common understanding, the necessity of giving up the indulgence of individual will when it conflicts with the public good. Hence municipal laws for regulating thoroughfare, and for the introduction and export of various articles of commerce, especially the products of agriculture. Every citizen is insured the right of way through all the streets, in the pursuit of business or pleasure; and he is protected by stringent laws from the dishonesty of those who would sell him tainted meat, or provisions at short weight. It is not in any view of sentimental philanthrophy or of ascetic restriction, but in the name of humanity and justice, that so many of our fellow-citizens, in all the walks of life, are urgent for similar prohibitions against the retail trade in liquid poison, the product of alcoholic distillation—the original noxious effects of which on the animal economy are still further increased by the addition of some of the most subtle and active poisons derived from other sources.

Individual caprice and heedlessness are checked in acts which conflict with the rights of the majority, in fact, of the public at large, as when a person would extend the front of his house beyond the regular line, or pile up goods or wares in the middle of the street. It would be well that some limitation should be put also to the height of the house, in order that a whole neighborhood and the passers-by may not be put in jeopardy, or suffer from the loss of limb and life itself by the fall of these lofty structures, which are neither dedicated to religion nor to any public use, but which seem to be merely monuments of the silly vanity of individuals. The exclusion of the cheerful and genial sunlight from the street, and the restricted ventilation produced by such lofty piles, might count for something, even though questions of this nature do not enter into the calculations of cost and profit by the first owners. Paving and draining and sewerage are also recognized parts of city police and sanitary legislation, to which all holders of property are made to contribute, for the public good as well as for their own personal benefit. Public convenience and public health are subserved by these means, the performance or which is insured by regularly appointed agents, and boards of health. Few will be found in the large cities of Europe and America to contest the propriety and wisdom of all these measures of public hygiène, to which must be added the procuring a suitable supply of pure water, although, in many smaller placcs, they may be, at first, thought to be uncalled for, and to involve an expenditure of money beyond the good to be obtained. It is seldom, however, that experience does not show the groundless nature of these objections, both in a sanitary and economical point of view. There are not wanting, indeed, persons in every country, Christian or Mohammedan, who claim, as one of their reserved rights, the privilege of having their senses of sight and smell assailed by emanations from all kinds of offal and garbage, and the stagnant water of gutters, as if to mark the difference between town and country, and, at the same time, their freedom from restrictive laws. There are also not a few who, with tastes akin to those of the preceding class, claim that their house is their castle, and that they have a right to exclude the air from it as carefully as if they were in a state of siege, and had been obliged to close every aperture through which an enemy's missile might find entrance.

Community of Interests.—State policy, isself, however little affinity it may seem to have to philanthropy and philosophy, is deeply concerned in the inculcation and enforcement of the true principles of public hygiene. The power of a state depends on the population, wealth, and productive industry, and on the cultivated intelligence of its people; trammels on all of which are created by whatever deteriorates the physical strength and the health of any portion of them. Permanent injury to the public health exerts, at the same time, an unfavorable influence on the social state; and hence poverty, with its frequent concomitants of hunger and the daily alternations of eager expectation of relief and of depression of the feelings, has ever been a promoter of secret and political disorganization. While philanthropy incites to more extended efforts for the relief and prevention of sufferings which are the result of a breach of the natural laws or those of health, expanded philosophy teaches that, although some classes in every city pay the heaviest penalties, yet there is no one class exempt from similar inflictions. The rich man, in his spacious mansion, has a direct personal interest in the health and domestic comfort of his poor neighbor ; and the more secluded and shut out from the world, in a dark court or alley, is this neighbor, the greater is this interest. His open windows will give entrance, not only to the refreshing breeze, but also to the poisoned air emanating from congregated beings in the confined lodgings, and from the unremoved refuse or offal adjacent. It is thus that Typhus Fever, beginning in the hovels of the poor, finds its way into the luxurious abodes of the rich. Were it necessary to continue in this line of argument, we might point to the importance of sanitary legislation for the employer or master manufacturer, as well as for the operatives and workmen. His real interest will not consist in obtaining from them the greatest possible amount of work from day to day, without reference to their having a due proportion of time for sleep, and of moderate recreation in the open air. Nor will it be good economy to stint these persons in the quantity of wholesome food which is necessary not merely to remove the cravings of hunger, but to renovate the body weakened by labor. The landlord who desires to have his houses always occupied by good paying tenants, will not be negligent of either their health or their morals. He will not speculate on the powers of endurance of human beings, when deprived of fresh air by residence in close, damp, and badly-ventilated rooms, and who are compelled to inhale an impure and vitiated air, the product of their own respiration, and the exhalations from the accumulated filth of cess-pools, and of yards choked up by offal. The inmates of such habitations are, necessarily, less fitted for labor and active employment of every kind; lose more time by sickness, and are carried off in larger proportion by death than those in more favorable hygienic conditions. Their nervous system is weakened in the functions of the senses and of the brain; and, even if intemperance should not add its baneful influence to their distress, they are more susceptible to the causes of moral disorders and the temptations to evil doing. Men, thus wearied and worn, depressed in body and in mind, and deprived of all the genial excitement from fresh air and light, and shut out from all the objects which might remind them of nature, under her more pleasing aspects, become careless of themselves, indifferent to the wants of their families, and regardless of the obligations contracted with employer and landlord, or with the administrators of the laws. They are unfitted for prolonged and regular labor. They are bad workmen, bad tenants, and unsafe neighbors. We shall conclude what is to be said of the benefits of a good sanitary system, both to the rich and the poor, by repeating that right royal sentiment of Prince Albert, on the occasion of his taking the chair at a meeting of the "Society for improving the Condition of the Working Classes." "Depend upon it," said the princely chairman, "that the interests of the often-contrasted classes are identical, and it is only ignorance which prevents their uniting to the advantage of each other."

Paving.—The sanitary reforms which have been carried out within the last ten or fifteen years in Great Britain, and those which are still in progress, following as they do a careful investigation of the evils and abuses to be corrected, enable us to speak with additional confidence of the importance and economy of sanitary measures to cities, and to adduce a large body of facts alike pertinent and convincing. Your reporter will content himself with introducing at this time some statements taken from a mass of evidence which he had previously collected for other purposes. To begin with *paving*, it might be sufficient to say that the evils from neglect of it are pointed out in most of the reports on the health of towns, but we cannot forbear from again adverting to the effects witnessed in London. Before the streets of that metropolis were paved, the inhabitants were as great sufferers from periodical fevers as those of the worst situated rural districts in our own country, and until underground drainage had been adopted to some extent, dysentery was common and largely fatal. Drawing on home experience, it has been found that in Philadelphia, the exemption of the inhabitants from intermittent and bilious remittent fevers has, with great uniformity, followed the paving of the streets. The space now called Dock street was, in the early days of the history of Philadelphia, a miry swamp, traversed by the sluggish stream Dock creek, on either side of which periodical fevers, of all grades, prevailed with a violence equal to those met with in the most sickly districts in distant States. The exposed surface having been paved, and the creek partly filled up and covered over, and made the line of a great culvert, no person residing there now has any apprehension of fevers, such as those that affected the former dwellers there. A like change from the operation of a similar cause has been wrought in the districts of Southwark, Kensington, aud Richmond. The change in the sanitary condition of Southwark is the more obviously due to paving and subsequent attention to scavengering, as the greater part of the drainage is on the surface, owing to the limited extent of sewers.

An important lesson is deduced from the history of the foundation of new cities, or the extension of the streets of old ones, viz.: that paving ought to precede the erection of houses, and drainage follow habitation at a very early period. A neglect of these two preliminary conditions for public health has been productive, in all ages, of a fearful waste of life; we say waste, because the deaths were readily preventable. Actually at this time the pavement of the seventy miles of streets in Boston furnishes a cheap protection to the inhabitants against the evils arising out of the constant presence and accumulation of town mud and filth, and other abominations which it would be impossible to remove from any ground not coated in this way. This is the more evident when we learn that for the length of seventy miles of streets, there are but twenty-five miles of sewers, many of which were some years ago one third to one half filled with mud. Baltimore is mainly indebted to street pavement for the drainage which is done at the surface, as the aggregate length of all the sewers ten years ago did not exceed two miles. One of the most remarkable examples of the beneficial change in the health of a city produced by paving its streets, is furnished in the history of Louisville, Kentucky, which from being called the grave-yard of the West, is now regarded as one of the most healthy cities of that extensive region. Intermittent fever was, as we learn from Dr. L. P. Yandell, a regular annual visitor, and occasionally a form of bilious fever prevailed, rivaling Yellow Fever in malignity, and threatening to depopulate the town. The citizens, awakened, after the fever of 1822, to a sense of their condition and to the means of mending it, set about a system of improvement, the chief feature of which was paving of the streets and filling up of the ponds. The change in the sanitary character of Louisville is the more noticeable, as it was brought about without the aid of subsoil drainage by sewers.

It has been truly said that fever loves the banks of rivers, the borders of marshes, the edges of stagnant pools ; it makes itself at home in the neighborhood of cess-pools and badly constructed drains, and takes especial delight in the incense of gully-holes. It should be added at the same time, that fever, at least of the periodical kind, will be prevented from showing itself by its favorite haunts being covered with a good pavement, so as to separate at once and permanently from the sun and air, the bed of moist putrefactive materials which ferment and give rise to the continual evolution of noxious gases. But the guardians of the public health must not relax their vigilance after the construction of suitable street pavements, for, unless there be enforcement of a regular system of scavengering, their surface will soon be covered with semi-fluid mud, and offal, and vegetable and animal refuse, which will represent too faithfully and fatally the banks of rivers, a marsh, or the edge of ponds, and the contents of cess-pools and gullies.

Cleansing of the Streets.—Cleansing of the streets, by a proper system of scavengering, is called for, both by the requirements of health and of comfort. The streets have been said, with justice, to be the reservoirs whence we are supplied with fresh air, and if it be impure in them, it is impure everywhere. It is not enough to prevent the access of foul air from untrapped and unwashed drains, but also from surface filth, and the remains of any kind accumulated in the streets. Further, continues the writer who makes these remarks, Mr. P. H. Holland, of Manchester, dirty streets cause dirty houses, dirty clothes, dirty persons; every one walking in them in wet weather carries into his house some portion of dirt, to increase the difficulty of domestic cleanliness. In dry weather the same effect is perhaps more powerfully produced by constant clouds of dust.

Economy of Street Cleaning.—The great obstacle to increased cleanliness of the streets, is the expense of frequent scavengering. Mechanical ingenuity has, within a few years past, obviated, in a considerable degree, this objection. Mr. Whitworth, the celebtated mechanic of Manchester, has perfected a sweeping machine, by means of which he is enabled to sweep the streets of that town three times as often as they used to be by hand, and at the same cost. In Birmingham, Leeds, London, and several other places, this machine has likewise been worked with success. In Liverpool, from some unexplained cause, it has not given equal satisfaction-

The expense of cleaning the streets and ash-bins, &c., is balanced by the sale of ashes and dust by the parishes of London. The experience of Edinburgh shows that, under proper officers, the daily cleaning of the city, and of its numerous courts and closes, is attainable at the moderate expense of ten thousand dollars a year. In Aberdeen, the work is done daily, at a profit to the city of a sum equal to three thousand dollars. In Hull, they have discovered that they can readily dispose of to small farmers—who find it their interest to collect it—the refuse from the houses, even in the courts and alleys, which are inaccessible to carts. Small streets, as well as courts and alleys, are apt to be neglected by the scavengers, and if any of these be unpaved, stagnant puddles are the consequence, and the atmosphere, necessarily close and confined in such spots, becomes still further deteriorated by the accumulations of refuse and filth, not to speak of the presence of open privies.

Sewered and Unsewered Districts compared.—In contrasting the effects on the health of the inhabitants of *sewered* with *unsewered* districts in the same town, we are met by the remarkable example of Ashton-under-Lyne in England, in which the duration of life is six years more in the former than in the latter portions. Equally marked results have been obtained from the sanitary records of Chorlton, a township of Manchester. While the mortality in the undrained streets amounts to four per cent., in the drained districts it is only two per cent.; and that we do not overrate the influence of drainage, is proved by the fact that some streets containing 3500 inhabitants, and exhibiting a mortality of 1 in 32 of the population, were elevated immediately after having obtained the benefit of sewerage to such a scale of health, that the deaths decreased to 1 in 50, or in other words, the deaths were diminished 20 a year out of every 110, even as a first effect of putting the streets in a proper condition as to sewerage. Other districts of Manchester give the same instructive lesson. In Liverpool it was ascertained that although the high mortality of 5.4 per cent. occurred in both sets of courts in that city, yet that more than 22 persons in every 100 of the undrained courts had serious cases of illness, while only 10 in 100 suffered in the same way in the drained districts. The sanitary history of every city contains evidence of the improvement of the public health following a good system of sewerage. Proof is also furnished in the contrast offered between the preferred and fashionable streets as we now find them, and the same spots before they had the benefit of paving and sewerage. In London, the west end of the city, and Westminster, the seats of the residences of the nobility, and where are found the courts of law and the two houses of Parliament, were once extensive marshes, nearly uninhabitable on account of the fevers which annually prevailed there. In Paris a regular system of sewerage has converted sickly and almost abandoned districts into those now known as the Faubourg Montmartre, the Chaussé d'Antin, and the Faubourg St. Honoré, which are remarkable for the business transacted in them, and the wealth of their inhabitants,

Rotherhithe, a district of London, on the south bank of the Thames, has been the favorite haunt of the cholera in successive periods of appearance of that disease from 1831–2 to 1854. Its sewerage was deplorably defective, being by open sewers connected with the river. Malignant cholera spread to a much greater extent on the line of open sewers than in the other poor and densely inhabited places. In other districts, we are told that the line of habitations, badly cleansed and suffering from defective drainage, formed the line of cholera cases in 1831–2. The reports of the medical inspectors, appointed by the Board of Health in London, in 1854, concur in showing that wherever cholera has become localized, it was found to be connected with obvious removable causes. Of these, the principal were the open ditches used in most instances as sewers, or receptacles of all descriptions of filth, and receiving the drainage of numerous privies. Generally speaking, the mortality from cholera was greatest in the lowest levels, owing, as may readily be supposed, to their imperfect drainage, and consequently to the greater humidity and impurity of the air of such places. The advantages that might be expected from greater elevation are lost however, by defective or inefficient drainage, as in the instance of the district of Kensal, in the parish of Chelsea, near London, if not now an integral part of the metropolis. This district, with the advantage of having at least 50 feet higher elevation than the rest of the parish, and an open airy situation, had a death-rate from epidemic disease, principally diarrhœa, nearly double that of any other district in the parish; although if we exclude epidemic disease, it is actually the healthiest of the Chelsea districts. The defective sanitary arrangement, on which this state of things depends, is described by Dr. Barclay, Medical Officer of Health for Chelsea, to be inefficient drainage, fecal fermentation, and the impregnation of the atmosphere with unwholesome emanations from foul drains, ditches, and cess-pools. It has been said that the course of Typhoid Fever in a town may be tracked by that of neglectod sewerage. In Croydon, a town not far from London, in consequence of a new but badly constructed system of drainage, there occurred "an alarming outbreak of Fever, (Typhoid), Diarrhœa, and Dysentery." And the relator, Dr. Letheby, adds, that Dr. Carpenter, of that town, informed him "that even now he can tell where the pipes are stopped, by the occurrence of Diarrhœa or Fever in the houses through which the foul gases are forced." Typhoid Fever has been represented to be a better test than even Diarrhœa of the sanitary state of a town.

The unhealthiness of an urban or suburban district, and its

liability to visitations of Fevers and Cholera, depend in no small degree on its low situation and its proximity to river-banks, or to stagnant water, and too commonly still on its imperfect drainage. It was said, in reference to the intimate relations between the activity of the disease, and the proximity of the river Thames, that two causes are at work in such a locality. First, increased humidity, and, secondly, and more especially, the large evaporating surface of foul water, by which noxious effluvia are continually given off, and poison, to a certain extent, the atmosphere through which they are diffused. On this point, the language held by Dr. Grainger, will properly find a place on the present occasion: "It is almost needless to point out," writes this gentleman, "that when the numerous sewers of a city reach the stream, one part of their contents widely mingling with a large body of water, undergoes solution, and thus presents a physical condition favorable to their subsequent escape into the atmosphere in the form of mephitic gases; whilst other portions, owing to the diminished velocity, sink to the bottom, near the edge of the river, and thus become deposited on the banks of putrid mud, which will at the next tide, being laid bare to the action of the sun and air, exhale poisonous effluvia." This writer adds, that some facts came to his knowledge, showing that it is precisely in those spots at the stream, which receive the principal body of sewerage, that Cholera especially ravages the population. We may add that it was so at Hamburg and at Berlin, in the latter of which cities open drains emptying their contents into the sluggish Spree, would be productive of still greater mischief. In Paris, the evils from this cause have been felt, and suggestions were made some years ago, and have been in a measure carried out, to construct two great tunnel sewers, one on each side of the Seine, to receive and transmit to some distance below the city all the sewerage of the different branch-sewers. A similar project is now discussed in London, so that the Thames may cease to be, as it has been for a long time past, the great common and open sewer of the metropolis. In Philadelphia and New York, reforms are called for in this matter, so that the mouths of the sewers, which discharge their contents into the rivers of these two cities, shall not be exposed at low tide, and give out poisonous effluvia, which either directly generate malignant Fevers, or serve as exciting causes on organisms predisposed by atmospherical extremes, such as high heat and humidity. Without involving ourselves in doctrinal questions as to the origin of Yellow Fever, we are sure of receiving, from all quarters, the admission of the general sameness of the localities of this disease, and that these are distinguished by their consisting, for the most part, of alluvial and made soil, and by their being deficient in suitable drainage and analogous means of preserving the surface dry and clear of accumulations of filth and the like decomposed organic remains What is said of the Yellow Fever in New Orleans will apply to other places in which it has committed its worst ravages, viz., that it attacks, generally, at first, the most susceptible, who live in the filthiest, worst-drained and paved, and worst-ventilated, and most crowded portions of the city. In Philadelphia, invariably from the first visitation of the Yellow Fever in 1699, to the last slight one in 1853, the history of the origin of the first appearance of the Fever is told in nearly the same language, viz., in Dock street, near the drawbridge, the former mouth of Dock Creek, in different parts of Water street, or at the water-side, or on one of the wharves, between Kensington on the north, and Southwark on the south end of the city. In 1699 it broke out in the vicinity of the dock at the end of Spruce street; and in 1853 on or near the wharf at the Delaware corner of South street—the two spots being less than three hundred yards apart. Near the latter of the two, the mouth of a large sewer was exposed at low tide, and the emanations from its imperfectly discharged contents left to poison the air around. In New York, a still worse state of things prevails, not only from the same cause, but from the slips and docks, especially on the East River, being made the receptacles for all kinds of offal and refuse, thrown into them from the wharves and the vessels.

Sewage and Sewer Gases.—The virulent and actively poisonous nature of the emanations from sewage, whether at the terminations of the sewers left exposed in the manner now described, or in the course of its passage under the streets of a city, from gully-holes or leaks in the public sewers, as well as in the private drains leading into these latter, have been investigated with considerable care of late years both in London and Paris. In the British metropolis, Drs. Barker and Letheby, the first in a paper in the *Sanitary Review and Journal of Public Health*, Vol. IV., the second in a *Report to the Commissioners of Sewers of the City of London*, have entered very fully and ably into the subject. Dr. Barker instituted a number of experiments on animals, with a view of showing the toxical effects of the chief gases in sewer emanations, viz., carbonic acid, sulphuretted hydrogen, and ammonia, or rather sulphide of ammonium. A mouse, exposed in a cage to the air of a cess-pool, within three inches of the surface, although it was well fed at intervals, died on the fifth day. Dogs thus exposed suffered from vomiting, diarrhœa, and febrile symptoms, rigors, restlessness, thirst, and loss of appetite. The gases above named were then experimented with separately. A puppy, exposed to less than two per cent. of sulpheretted hydrogen in the common air, was destroyed in two minutes and a half, without a struggle, and so small a proportion as 0.428 per cent. killed another in an hour. A dog, exposed to 0.205 per cent. of this gas, was affected within a minute by tremors, and fell on his side. The action of the heart became irregular, and within four minutes the respiration had apparently ceased, but after awhile was renewed. After one hour and thirty-eight minutes the dog was removed from the box containing air mixed with sulpheretted hydrogen as above. The respirations, which had, previously, at one time—three quarters of an hour from the beginning of the experiment—been 112 and even 120 in a minute, became suddently stertorous, as in apoplexy. On the removal of the dog the respirations were stertorous, the limbs rigid, and the head was drawn backwards: the animal died nine hours and thirty-eight minutes after the commencement of the experiment. A second dog, similarly exposed, suffered at first, but soon revived, and at the end of five hours, was removed without exhibiting any morbid effect. Another was attacked with tremblings and diarrhœa after breathing the gas; a fourth with all the appearances of intoxication. Ammonia and its salts produced what Dr. Richardson, in his Essay on the Causes and Coagulation of the Blood, considers to be unmistakably typhoid symptoms. The minute quantity of 0.056 per cent. or 56 parts of sulphuretted hydrogen in a thousand of common air, is sufficient to produce serious symptoms—eructations, tremors, rapid and irregular respiration, extraordinary rapidity of the pulse, and diarrhœa. The inhalation of carbonic acid in small proportions was followed by diarrhœa. Dr. Barker arrived at the following conclusions, which may be received as a fair expression of the facts:

"The symptoms which have been noticed as resulting from the inhalation of sulpheretted hydrogen, sulphide of ammonium, and carbonic acid, are sufficient to account for the effects arising from cess-pool effluvia, without seeking for any further product from such emanations. Comparing the experiments with cess-pool air with those in which separate gases were employed, the inference seems clear to my mind, that the symptoms arising from the inhalation of cess-pool atmosphere were due mainly to the presence of a small amount of sulpheretted hydrogen, which gas was always present. If the experiments with the cess-pool air be placed side by side with those in which sulpheretted hydrogen, in the proportion of 0.056 per cent. was administered by inhalation, the analogy between the two sets of results will be sufficiently unmistakable."

Before inquiring into the nature, and the effects on the animal economy of sewage gases, Dr. Letheby examines the *nature of sewage* itself—as far as observed by this writer, in reference to what is met with in England. The matters to be dealt with in the public sewers of every town and city are very complex, for they are composed not only of the solid and liquid ejecta of the population, but also of the fluid refuse of every branch of industry. They consist of the filth of kitchens, laundries, and dye-houses; the drainings from stables, slaughter-houses, and the public markets; the various liquid impurities of trade and manufactories; and the washings of the streets and alleys; all of which, with the ejecta of the inhabitants and a large quantity of water, compose the sewage of towns. In Paris and the French towns generally, and in our American ones, a difference prevails in their sewage from that of London and other towns in England, in the circumstance of the small quantity of human ejecta which is conveyed by private sewers into the public ones in France and the United States. Altogether, it may be said, that the ejecta of the inhabitants of London and the washings of the streets daily, furnish about 233 tons of solid matter to the sewage, of which 152.6 tons are of dry matter, and 293.6 of moist, and these with the trade refuse, are diluted with about 84¾ million gallons of water. It has been estimated, as data for part of the preceding calculations, that 2 to 2½ ounces of dry solid matter are contained in the excrements *per diem* of each member of the population. Another mode of estimating the composition of sewerage is founded on the analytical results of its examination at different times and places. These show that the sewage discharge by day is richer in solid material than the night sewage is; and that there are considerable differences in this respect between the contents of sewers situated in different quarters of the city. "Taking the average of all the results obtained in the examination of the metropolitan sewers, it may be concluded that the sewage which flows into the Thames contains about 90¼ grains of solid matter in the gallon; of which about 29¾ are suspended, and 60½ dissolved: there being about 15 grains of organic matter in each of these constituents." "The mineral constituents of sewer-water are chiefly carbonate of lime and common salt, with small proportions of the alkaline sulphates and phosphates. They are derived from urine and from the water supply. The mineral part of the insoluble matter consists almost entirely of the *debris* of the streets, and detritus of wheels and horse-shoes. Their amount is about 15 grains per gallon; which, in the aggregate, is as near as possible 81 tons per day for the whole of the metropolis, or 19 for the city." "Then, of the total amount of 485.5 tons of solid matter contained in the sewage of one day, about 152.60 tons are the ejecta of the inhabitants; 81.08 tons the pulverized granite and iron on the roads; 102.04 the saline matter contained in the water supply; and the residue, 152.78 tons, is from trade and manufactures. The total amount of organic matter in all this is about 215.14 tons; of which half is in a state of solution, and the rest is suspended.

"The physical properties of the sewage are peculiar, for when it is examined under the microscope, it is found that the clear supernatant part contains a large quantity of amorphus organic matter, with the filaments of various fungi. It swarms with animal life, as beaded *spirulina*, *vibriones*, and *monads;* and soon after exposure to air the higher forms of infusoria appear, as *paramecium*, *vorticella*, *rotifera*, &c. Besides which it contains small particles of animal and vegetable tissues, as the fibres of cotton, wool, &c." "The mineral part is composed of the *débris* of the streets, as particles of granite, flint, and carbonate of lime, with a large quantity of the black sulphuret of iron. When the sewage has a very unpleasant odor, and is charged with sulphureted hydrogen, it never exhibits much sign of animal or vegetable life, notwithstanding that it contains an abundance of decaying organic matter. This is the case with the foul contents of the nearly stagnant sewers."

The putrefactive decomposition of sewage is noticed by Dr. Letheby. Looking at the enormous quantity of organic matters contained in sewage, and its minute subdivision, proportion of water, and temperature, it is not surprising that its decomposition should be attended with the evolution of a large amount of noxious gas, or that it should at once take on the putrefactive change, and begin to evolve foul gases, before it enters the sewers. "Under ordinary circumstances, the solid excrements do not ferment in less than three or four days, but here the catalytic influences are so strong, that putrefaction begins at once, and it is always of the same kind as that already in progress in the old sewer matter. This tendency to accelerate and direct the decomposition is very remarkable. Its power lasts for weeks after the sewage has ceased to ferment, or it will operate immediately in all kinds of organic substances. Blood, sugar, feces, urine, and other fermentable bodies are rapidly changed by it; and they evolve compounds of a most offensive character. Common sugar, instead of being fermented into alcohol, is converted into lactic acid, which smells like putrid pig's-wash; then it passes into butyric acid, and gives hydrogen and carbonic acid, with the odor of rancid butter and human perspiration."

Dr. Letheby points out the important part which the oxygen of the atmospheric air performs in the sewers, by giving birth to mineral products, as water, carbonic acid, the sulphates, phosphates, and nitrates, which are the final products of decay. "Its influence, therefore, is most salutary, and ought not to be disregarded. Experiment has also shown that the oxydizing power of the air is promoted by water, by porous substances, and by the fixed alkalies." Dr. L. ascertained that it is the solid part of the sewerage which continues to ferment and keep up the putrefactive action for months, evolving large quantities of ammonia, sulphuretted hydrogen, marsh gas, and carbonic acid. It is the sedimentary matter which is the chief cause of the effluvium, and to this the writer afterwards directs attention.

The Nature of the Sewer Gases.—Dr. Letheby judiciously precedes his observations on this subject by the observation, that little can be really done in the way of providing a remedy for the sewer miasms, until something is definitely known of their nature and composition. He has endeavored to procure the knowledge wanted, by three sets of investigations, viz.: "1. From inquiries into the composition of the gases dissolved in sewage; 2. From an analysis of the gases evolved during its putrefaction; and 3. From an examination of the sewer air itself." The clear liquid of sewage, when heated, evolves all the gases which were held in solution. These consist of carbonic acid, sulphuretted hydrogen, ammonia, marsh gas (carburetted hydrogen), and nitrogen. Their quantity varies from about 32 to 76 cubic inches per gallon; and the proportion of carbonic acid varies from 36 to 72 per cent.; the sulphuretted hydrogen from 0.9 to 3.1. A fact, full of significance, in relation to the condition of that river in its course through London, is stated here. It is, that Thames water, near to the shore at low tide, contains the same ga[illegible]arly the same proportion. It was observed that these gases are abundantly evolved wherever the sewerage becomes stagnant, or nearly so. From the thick slushy matter in one sewer (that of Catharine-wheel alley) the carburetted hydrogen, among other gases, bubbled up in such quantities that it could be ignited with ease, and would thus set fire to the neighboring bubbles and produce a sheet of flame that would extend for some distance along the surface of the sewage. "The gas contained 63 per cent. of inflammable air; 17.6 of carbonic acid; 14.1 of nitrogen, and 0.2 of sulphuretted hydrogen. The amount of ammonia contained in the liquid of sewage is also considerable. It ranges from 3 to 15 grains in the gallon of ordinary sewage, and from 15 to 41 in that of nearly stagnant sewers. In addition to all these, there are other volatile compounds which have not yet been isolated—compounds which give to the sewage its peculiar odor, and which Dr. Letheby surmises may also cause its poisonous action. Looking at the experiments of Dr. Baker, previously noticed, we may doubt the necessity of searching for other and unknown toxical agents to give rise to morbid phenomena which are already strictly ascribable to known gases. The English writer made experiments similar to those performed thirty years ago in Paris by Gaultier de Claubry, which show the great diminution of oxygen, the increase of nitrogen, and the evolution of sulphuretted hydrogen in sewer air. He was able to condense the organic vapor which rose from the sewer air, as had been done by the French commissioner appointed to report on the cleaning and purifying of the public sewers of Paris, at the time just mentioned, and of which Parent-Duchatelet was a member. The liquid thus obtained had a very disagreeable and putrid and ammoniacal odor, like that of bad sewage.

On the subject of the *properties of the sewage gases and their effects on the animal system*, we gather some interesting facts from Dr. Letheby's Report. He begins with sulphuretted hydrogen, which experiments, performed many years ago by Dupuytren and Thenard, show to be eminently poisonous, even in very minute quantities. Horses are killed by an atmosphere containing one part of it in 250 of the air; but much less is hurtful if it be breathed for any length of time. It is on record, that the men who were engaged in cutting through the bed of the river, for the construction of the Thames tunnel, suffered severely from the effects of the gas, although the proportion of it in the air was hardly to be discovered by lead paper, and could not, therefore, have exceeded one part in 100,000. It is true that it sometimes came in gushes from the fissures of the mud, but the quantity was rarely sufficient to be recognizable by its odor. Strong and robust men were, however, reduced to a state of extreme exhaustion by breathing it for a few months, and several of them died from this cause. The symptoms with which they were affected were giddiness, nausea or actual sickness of stomach, and great debility. The men became emaciated, lost their appetites, and fell into a state of low fever, from which, in several instances, they did not recover. Chloride of lime and other prophylactics were used, but the evil did not entirely cease until the tunnel was opened from end to end, and free ventilation established. Dr. Taylor mentions another remarkable instance of the same kind of poisoning, which occurred in the summer of 1857, at Clayton Moor, near Whitehaven, where there is a row of small cottages built on the refuse slag of some neighboring iron furnaces. In the course of two days, in the month of June, thirty of the inhabitants, all of whom had been for some time previously annoyed by an offensive smell, were made seriously ill by it. In a family of seven persons, consisting of a husband and wife, and five children, who had retired to rest in their usual health, two were found dead the next morning, and the others were in a state of insensibility. "Before the day was over, another of them died, and in the course of the week a fourth. In the second case, a strong, healthy man came home from his night-work, and went to bed; but an hour had hardly elapsed when he also was found dead. And in a sixth instance, a child was taken ill in the morning and was a corpse at night." In an inquiry instituted on the occasion, in order to discover the cause of the mischief, Dr. Taylor came to the conclusion that it was the sulphuretted hydrogen, generated by the action of water on the refuse slag upon which the houses were built. If the explanation be a correct one, the case is a remarkable instance of the poisonous action of this gas, for the test of lead paper failed to show the presence of the poison except in mere traces, that is, in quantities which could not have been greater than one part in 100,000 of the air. "These experiments and observations show that sulphuretted hydrogen gas is a powerful narcotic poison; that in a concentrated state it kills immediately, as with the energy of prussic acid. In a more dilute form, it causes death by lingering stupor, and when more diluted still, so as hardly to be discovered by the odor, it prostrates the vital powers, and produces a low fever, which may end fatally."

"*Carbonic acid* is also produced by the decay of organic matters. It is found in the air of sewers to the extent of 0.5 to 2.3 per cent., and the gases evolved from the sewage itself contain about 19 per cent. of it. If the gas has been produced at the expense of the oxygen of the air, as happens in sewers and crowded rooms, the effects are more strongly marked, for under these circumstances as little as three per cent. will quickly destroy life, and even the proportion of from 1.5 to 2 per cent. will cause almost immediate distress and feelings of suffocation, with often giddiness and headache, and a sense of weight and throbbing of the temples. This is sometimes followed by a slight delirium, and then by an irresistible desire to sleep, the stupor of which passes slowly into coma."

Ammonia is another constituent of the sewer air, and is a product of putrefaction. It is known by its peculiar odor and alkaline reaction. It is lighter than the common air in the proportion of 590 to 1000. "When ammonia is inhaled in a concentrated state, it produces immediate asphyxia; when it is somewhat diluted with air, its action is chiefly on the lungs; and when it is more diluted still, and is breathed for a considerable time, it liquefies the corpuscles of the blood, and produces the symptoms of typhoid fever." These observations are confirmed by Dr. Barker's experiments. Dr. Richardson, already quoted, in the same sense, finds, from experiment, that the continued action of ammoniacal gas, even when it is largely diluted with air, is peculiarly injuri- to the animal economy: the tongue becomes dry and dark, there is an involuntary action of the muscles, varying from mere twitching to violent convulsions; there are insensibility, extreme sensitiveness to sound, obscurity of sight, and ultimately, if matters are pushed far enough, death by coma. The state of the organs after death tends to the same conclusion. The blood is dark and fluid; the serous membranes show petechial spots, and the tissues are softened. "But," adds Dr. Letheby, "there is another property of ammonia which is more dangerous still: it is that of conveying the less volatile products of putrefaction into the air. In all probability it is the purveyor of the miasms of infected districts, as it is known to have the fetid compounds of animal and vegetable decomposition. It was the agent which gave validity to the putridities of the Thames during the hot weather, and it is the medium by which the more offensive matters of coal gas are held in suspension. Nor is it less powerful by by diffusing the sweet odors of plants and the subtle constituents of many perfumes. It may, therefore, act for good as well as for evil.

"*The volatile* compounds of ammonia, with carbonic acid

and sulphuretted hydrogen, are also injurious. The first act like the alkali itself, and the second like sulphuretted hydrogen. I have found that one part of hyposulphate of ammonia in 1000 of air will kill birds almost instantly, and one in 500 will kill rabbits."

"*Light carburetted hydrogen*, or *marsh gas*, is also found in the atmosphere of sewers, but it rarely occurs in such proportion as to be dangerous; now and then, however, it accumulates, as it does in coal mines, and becomes explosive." Miners are often obliged to work in an atmosphere containing from 8 to 10 per cent. of the gas, but they experience no ill effects from it, until the proportion rises to about 20 per cent., and then they feel giddy, with a sense of weight upon the forehead

"*Coal gas* is likewise present in the sewers; it is not found there, but escapes from the street mains. The quantity which is let loose in this manner is enormous Gas consumers say that from 12 to 35 per cent. of all the gas manufactured in London is lost. Now supposing that of this, the leakage amounts to five per cent., which my friend, Mr. Wright, informs me is about the quantity, then as much as 386,400,000 cubic feet of gas escape into the public ways of the metropolis every year, or rather more than a million cubic feet every day; and in the city it amounts to about 25,000,000 cubic feet *per annum*, or nearly 70,000 cubic feet per day. Most of this must find its way into the sewers, and therefore is a matter of some importance. The chief constituents of coal gas are hydrogen, and light carburetted hydrogen. The former amounts to about 40 per cent. of the gas, and the latter to 45. The other constituents are about 7 per cent. of carbonic oxide, 2 of nitrogen 1 of carbonic acid, and 5 of the condensable hydrocarbons, besides which, there are always traces of ammonia, bisulphuret of carbon, and coal tar. The principal danger from this gas is its inflammability, and its property of forming an explosive mixture with atmospheric air." "Dr. Taylor has attested the record of seven cases of death from the action of coal gas, and it is probable that the air was not charged with more than 8 or 9 per cent. of it in any one of them."

Dr. Letheby cannot speak with certainty of the *organic* vapor which is contained in sewer gases, "except that it is a matter in a state of active decomposition; and experience has long since decided that matter in this condition has power to disturb the equilibrium of other organic molecules, and to propagate to them its own state of decay. When this occurs in the living animal body, it is productive of the most terrible consequences. Our ignorance of the nature of this organic vapor is not surprising, when we consider that we are equally uninformed of the composition of the subtle miasms and putridities which abound in the air of infected districts, and in the vapors of organic decomposition." "Sometimes these miasms are colorless, but in the case of the sewer gases, it is the organic vapor which gives them their peculiar smell, for when the sulpheretted hydrogen is entirely removed, there are still the characteristic stinks which have been so accurately described by Parent-Duchatelet."

"*What are the dangers of the Complex Sewer Gases themselves?* Experience has shown that they are of two kinds, namely: the dangers which are incidental to the poisonous action of the gases; and those which arise from their explosive property." Observation has proved that these gases are among the most active poisons. Passing over a description of the acute forms of poisoning by them when inhaled in their undiluted state, it may be stated, as most german to the present inquiry, that when these gases are much diluted with atmospheric air, they produce a general prostration of the vital powers. "The appetite fails; the bowels become disturbed; diarrhœa of a chronic character sets in;

and the sufferer is either worn out by exhaustion, or he falls into a state of low fever, from which it is difficult to raise him."

Dr. Letheby gives additional point to this part of the subject by mentioning a few cases of chronic poisoning in which the effects were produced by the inhalation of very small quantities of sewer miasm. We cannot forbear from repeating his narrative, under a belief of their extreme appositeness to the immediate purposes of this report, and for the lessons of caution which they furnish. One of the most remarkable instances of this is recorded by M. D'Arcet. He states that there was a small lodging in Paris, consisting of a bed-room and ante-room, which had been successively tenanted by three vigorous young men, each of whom died within a few months of his occupying the place. D'Arcet was requested to examine the rooms, and ascertain the cause of the evil. He found that a pipe from a privy in the upper floor ran down by the side of the wall near to the head of the bed where the inmates slept. The pipe was unsound, and the wall was damp from leakage of the soil into it; but there was no perceptible smell in the room when D'Arcet examined it; nevertheless he had no doubt that the deaths of the former occupants were referable to the emanations from the wall. The pipe was therefore repaired, and from that time the unwholesomeness of the place was cured. Again, in August, 1831, twenty-two boys living at a boarding-school in Clapham, near London, were suddenly seized with alarming symptoms of irritation of the stomach and bowels, with twitchings of the muscles of the arms and excessive prostration of strength. Another boy had been similarly attacked three days before, and he died in twenty-five hours; one of the others died in twenty-three hours. A suspicion of accidental poisoning naturally arose, and the various utensils and articles of food used by the family were examined, but nothing of a deleterious nature was found. The only circumstance which appeared to explain the accident was, that two days before the first child was taken ill, a foul cess-pool had been opened, and the matter of it diffused over a garden adjoining to the children's play-ground. This was considered to be the cause of the disease, and the opinion was formed not only by the medical attendants, but also by Drs. Latham, Chambers, and Pearson, who personally examined the whole of the particulars. The third instance to which I shall refer is of more recent date, and has been a subject of considerable discussion. In the month of August, 1852, an attempt was made to drain the town of Croydon by means of small stoneware pipes, which were not only of insufficient size, but were imperfectly cemented together. The consequence was, that a large quantity of the sewage escaped into the earth, and drained away to the neighboring ditches. This became a subject of great annoyance, and in a short time it produced an alarming outbreak of Fever, Diarrhœa, and Dysentry. In the report from the Poor Law Commissioners on the sanitary condition of the laboring population of Great Britain, there are many examples of the morbific action of sewer and cess-pool gases. There is one case which is remarkable for its significance. "On the north side of a street in Derby there are fifty-four houses, all of the same description, and inhabited by the same class of persons. Six of these houses in the very centre of the row became the abodes of fever, and of sixteen persons attacked with the disease, five died. The fever was nowhere else in the row, and on inquiry it was found that these, and these only, were exposed to the action of sewer gases, and the miasms from cess-pool matter which had soaked into the soil."

It is impossible to carry the observations and experiments of Drs. Barker and Letheby in our minds without our comprehending the noxious agencies by which obstinate and often fatal diseases of the digestive organs, and low fevers, are produced in those parts of a town where the inhabitants are continually exposed to the operation of the gases above mentioned. These arise from vegetable and animal matter in decay and decomposition, from obstructed gutters, open drains, or from cess-pools, and the mouths and gully-holes of sewers, and accidental openings in these latter. Even when not directly poisoned by the continued inhalation of a corrupt atmosphere always charged with these gaseous poisons, the people thus exposed acquire such a predisposition—have their vital energies so much reduced—are primed as it were—that a slight change in the ordinary conditions of the atmosphere, or diminution of their accustomed food, serves as a spark to ignite into febrile fire their weakened and susceptible frames.

On the means of remedying the sewer miasms, or of preventing the offensive and toxical effects of the emanations from sewers, we cannot do better than introduce that portion of Dr. Letheby's report, the title of which was furnished in a preceding page. His manner of treating the subject gives it a freshness and value that cannot fail to be acceptable even after the interesting report of Dr. Van Bibber. At any rate, coming directly in our line of practical precept in all that relates to sewerage and sewage, we have not hesitated to apply it to our own purposes.

"THE REMEDY FOR THE SEWER MIASMS.—This is the great question which you have submitted to me for consideration, and the preceding facts show clearly enough that it is an important question. I am far from thinking, with your engineer, that the mischief occasioned by sewer gases is not of such magnitude as to be worth a remedy that may cost sixpence a head to the population; nor do I believe that if you had temporized with the matter, and had yielded to the demand on the part of the public, to close up the ventilating gratings, which are now so offensive, and had thus turned the foul gases into the house-drains, the nuisance would have been regarded simply as a domestic evil, for which the cure was to be sought privately and individually by those who felt the annoyance; in fact, such a proceeding would have been unworthy of the trust which is reposed in you as the custodians of the public health, for it would have been a matter of life or death to the great bulk of the community.

"At all times attempts have been made to destroy or neutralize the offensive products of decomposition; and the simplest way of doing it has been by the use of another secret—a perfume of volatile oil, which would cover or mask the offensive body. These were the correctives employed in religious worship. They entered into the composition of the ointments of the high priest and the incense of the altar, and to this day they have enjoyed a reputation and general popularity which they have not deserved, for their action is not on the putrid product, but merely on the sense of smell, which they blunt to the action of the offensive vapor. In the middle ages, when the plague, the black death, and sweating sickness, and pestilential fever desolated the cities of Europe, immense importance was attached to the use of perfumes; fumigations, with costly spice and rich-smelling Oriental drugs, were largely used in the houses of the rich, but with no good effect. The ancients also knew the value of fire as a disinfectant; and they also made use of the fumes of burning sulphur.

"But the right knowledge of the action of disinfectants and deodorizers dates from a very recent period, for so late as the year 1773, Guyton Morveau, one of the best chemists of France, thought that the vapors of muriatic acid were the most powerful of disinfectants; and later still, in the year 1803, Dr. Carmichael Smith obtained a grant of £5000 from Parliament, for a suggestion which is nearly valueless, namely, the employment of the fumes of nitrous acid. Chlorine gas was discovered by Scheele in 1774, and soon afterwards its disinfecting properties were noticed by Berthollet, but its use cannot be dated farther back than the present century, when Guyton Morveau and Dupuytren first pointed out the great value of it as a disinfectant; and even then it was not generally employed; in fact, its present popularity dates only from the time that chloride of lime has been largely manufactured for bleaching purposes. Within the last twenty years almost all the refuse products of the arts, and a great number of special compounds, have been recommended for the deodorization of sewage, &c. . They all act in one of two ways; they either give stability to the organic matter, and so check its tendency to decay, or they operate on the putrid vapors, and destroy their offensive properties. This they do, either by fixing the effluvium, and forming compounds which are inert, or by breaking up the putrid molecule and changing its nature, or by expediting the process of decay, and hurrying it on to the last stage of oxydation.

"Those substances which give stability to organic matter are properly called *anti-septics* or *anti-putrescents*. They have always been more popular than any of the second class of deodorizers, because of their importance in the arts. Salt, sugar, vinegar, creosote, and the empyreumatic oils of wood, peat, coal, &c., are examples of this class. So also are chloride of zinc, sulphate of copper, and corrosive sublimate, substances which have been respectively patented by Sir William Burnett, Mr. Margary, and Mr. Kyan. Alum and the astringent matter of many vegetables have likewise been used for ages as the means of preserving gelatinous tissues in the form of leather. None of these, however, except the chloride of zinc, is applicable to the case before us, and that operates more as a deodorizer than an anti-putrescent. In fact, as I have already stated, the matters of sewage are always in a state of decomposition, and cannot, therefore, be treated with much advantage, unless the anti-septics are applied to them before they enter the sewers; and this, I need not say, is altogether impracticable. Even in Paris, where there are special contrivances for such a purpose, it fails, because of its utter impracticability.

"Of the second class of substances, namely, the *deodorizers* and *disinfectants*, there are many which deserve notice.

"Those which combine with the putrid gases and fix them into involatile form, are the metallic oxyds and their salts, as chloride and sulphate of zinc; acetate and nitrate of lead; sulphate, muriate and pyrolignate of iron; impure muriate of manganese; the refuse of bleaching works; common alum; the fixed alkalies; and the salts of lime and magnesia. Most of these compounds unite with sulpheretted hydrogen and ammonia of sewage, and so far, therefore, they remove the unpleasant smell of it, but they do not touch the organic vapors. Besides which, they are difficult to apply, and are very costly. In fact, putting aside all the working expenses that would attend their use, the mere cost of the deodorizers alone would range from £20,000 to upwards of £1,000,000 per annum for the city sewage, and from £1,000,000 sterling to £48,000,000 for the sewage of the whole of London. This, together with the insufficiency of their power as deodorizers, and the difficulty of applying them while the sewage is within the sewer, deprives them of all practical utility. That power which they possess, namely, the power of coagulating a great part of the soluble matter of sewage, and favoring the precipitation of the insoluble, can only be applied with any chance of success after the sewage has left the sewers; and, even then, there are but two of them, namely, lime and the superphosphate of lime with magnesia, that can be used with advantage.

"Of the second class of disinfectants, those which act chemically on the volatile matter, and break them up, so as to form new compounds, which are inert, the most important are chlorine, chloride of lime, hypochlorous acid, sulphurous acid, and nitrous acid. The first three of these, namely, chlorine and its oxy-compounds, operate by abstracting hydrogen from the putrid vapors, and perhaps, also, by decomposing water, and setting the oxygen free to destroy the miasm. The power is remarkably great, as may be seen by the action of chlorine or chloride of lime on ordinary sewage. Eight grains of chloride of lime, or less than an ounce of the solution of chlorine, will completely deodorize a gallon of sewage; and the diffusion of a little chlorine through the worst kind of sewer gases, is sufficient instantly to deprive them of their offensive odor. Nevertheless chloride of lime is a costly agent. If it be used in the proportion of only eight grains to the gallon, it will cost nearly £57,000 a year for the deodorization of the city sewage, and nearly £237,000 for the sewage of all London. As for the gas itself, it is almost impossible so to apportion and manage the diffusion of it in the sewers as not to have the chlorine or the sewer gases in excess.

"Sulphurous acid and nitrous acid are still less manageable, and besides that they are costly, and not nearly as powerful in their action as chlorine. Like chlorine, however, they disorganize the putrid molecules and decompose the hydrosulphuric compounds, and fix ammonia; but like it also they are powerful irritants, and could scarcely be let loose into the sewers without danger to the workmen.

"The last of the disinfectants are those which expedite the process of decay, to combine with oxygen, and to become inert. Of this class there are two members, namely, those which act chemically, and supply oxygen, of themselves, to the offensive compounds, and those which merely facilitate oxydation by their physical properties. The manganates and permanganates of potash are the best examples of the first class, and contain a large proportion of oxygen, which they freely give the putrid organic matter, and so destroy it. These compounds have been patented by Mr. Condy, of Battersea, and he supplies them in a state of solution of various strengths. That which I have used in my experiments contained nearly six per cent. of the permanganate, and could be supplied at a shilling a gallon. One hundred and fifty drops of it were sufficient to deodorize a gallon of ordinary sewage; but the disadvantage of it is, that it has no power to destroy the foul gases which have already escaped into the sewer air. Besides this, the cost of the material, even if it were used in proportion of 150 grains to the gallon, would be about £753,000 a year for the city sewage, or more than three millions per annum for that of the whole metropolis. Looking, however, merely at the chemistry of the subject, it must be admitted that Mr. Condy's solution is a powerful and valuable disinfectant.

"The second of this class of disinfectants are the agents which promote oxydation by a physical property, that is by bringing the putrid matters into contact with atmospheric oxygen. There are three of them, namely, fire, water, and porous solids. The first effects the change by active combustion, and the others by the slower process of oxydation, which is called eremacausis or slow burning. All of them, however, are complete in their action, and are under different circumstances more or less manageable and useful.

"The value of fire as a disinfectant was known and has been

recognized since the remotest time. The sacrificial altars of early nations were the rude methods by which the agent was employed; and so fully did the ancients believe in its salutary action, that in times of pestilence it was often resorted to as the only effective means of purifying the atmosphere. In the popular mind there has always been a notion that the plague of London was exterminated by the great fire. Powerful, however, as the agent is, it does not appear to be applicable to the destruction of the sewer gases, notwithstanding that the use of it for such a purpose has always been a favorite idea with every new commission to sewers, and is the basis of most of the amateur schemes of the present day. Mr. Bazalgette has stated, in his evidence before the House of Commons, that putting aside all the difficulties for controlling the course of the air, in the main channel of the sewers, and stopping the leakage from the thousands of openings in the street closets and drains, the mere cost of fuel for the furnaces would not be less than £80,000 a year, and perhaps it might reach to upwards of £200,000.

"The destruction of the sewer miasms by the agency of water is not quite so unmanageable, and has therefore received attention from many of the leading engineers of the present day. Mr. Bazalgette says of it, that it is the best and the only available means of purifying the sewers. As to its salutary action there can be no doubt, for its power as a disinfectant in the presence of atmospheric air is manifested in every river in the kingdom. Wheresoever the putrid refuse of a town mixes with a large volume of fresh water, there the process of oxydation is quickly carried out, and the offensive matters are rendered innocuous. Even the river Thames, except at a peculiarly dry and hot season, finds within itself a means of purification which is quite equal to the contaminating influence of the soluble organic matter that flows into it. This is effected by the physical power which water possesses of transferring oxygen from the atmosphere to the putrid products, and this is so great that it will even destroy the soluble organic constituents of ordinary sewage without further dilution with water. I cannot inform you very accurately what quantity of water is necessary for the purpose of disinfection. Already there is a daily supply of about thirty-one gallons to each of the inhabitants of this metropolis. But this is evidently not sufficient to cleanse the sewers, for, independently of the existence of a putrid atmosphere, there is the stronger evidence of their foulness and the condition of the sewage which is discharged after a heavy fall of rain. And even if it could be determined precisely what amount of water would effect the purpose, there is still the difficulty of distributing it so as to scour out all the channels: for this could not be accomplished without special contrivances for delivering the water at the head of every drain. I do not therefore see much prospect of success in this mode of dealing with the subject.

"The last means of destroying the offensive matter is by the agency of porous solids; and this may be applied either to the sewage itself, or to the gases which are evolved from it. The best examples of such an agent are common clay and charcoal. Both of them operate in the same way, namely, by condensing the putrid vapors within their pores and upon the surface, so as to cause them to unite with atmospheric oxygen, and produce in fact a species of slow combustion, by which the miasms are gradully consumed. To effect this, however, there must be a free access of atmospheric air. Hence it is these substances have but a limited power of deoxydation where they are mixed with a liquid sewage, or are so overcharged with water as to be incapable of absorbing oxygen.

"Every one is familiar with the deodorizing power of common earth; in fact, the grave-yards of every city testify to the enormous quantities of organic matter that can be disposed of through its agency, and no one who has witnessed the rapid deodorizing power of clay when sewage or night-soil is distributed upon the land, can doubt its efficacy. The Chinese have long taken advantage of this power, for they mix night-soil with one third of its weight of fat marl, and knead it into cakes, which are common articles of commerce. In practice also, it is found that a ton of clay will deodorize about three tons of the solid matter of sewage. But, powerful as is this action, it is not applicable to liquid sewage. Even in the case of charcoal, which is a much more energetic deodorizer than common clay, the power is speedily lost when it is mixed with fluid refuse. Dr. Hofman found that four cubic feet of charcoal began to lose their power of deodorization when about seventy-eight gallons, or rather more than three times their bulk, of the sewage had passed through them. Mr. Blythe's experiments are to the same effect. To this I may add that the cost of this mode of deodorization would be upwards of £230,000 a year for the city sewage. The remedy would be but imperfect, to say nothing of the fact that it would contribute largely to the solid matter already in the sewers.

"The most effective way of using charcoal as a deodorizer, is to take advantage of its power of absorbing the putrid miasms when they are in a vaporous condition. This power is remarkably great. It was noticed by Sausure as far back as 1814, that charcoal took from 75.90 times its bulk of various gases. Count Morozzo had also observed the same fact, and had directed attention to it; and later still, Messrs. Allen and Pepys found that different kinds of charcoal had different powers of absorption; and yet it is only very recently that we have been well informed in this matter, and we owe our knowledge of it to the researches of Dr. Stenhouse, who in 1853 had his attention directed to the fact, that when dead bodies of large animals are covered with a layer of charcoal, they putrefy without evolving any unpleasant odor, notwithstanding that they are kept for many months.

" *Charcoal as an Air-Filter.*—These results suggested the use of charcoal as a respirator and an air-filter, and soon after Dr. Stenhouse proposed it as a purifier of the foul gases which escape from the street gullies, the sewers, ventilators, and the drains of private houses. One of his air-filters is in action in the justice-room of the Mansion House, and another is in the justice-room of Guildhall, and Dr. Stenhouse reports that their operations have been successful and continuous for a long time. I have myself repeated some of Dr. Stenhouse's experiments during the last twelve months, and have ascertained that the offensive gases from a close cess-pool are completely deodorized by passing them through a small box containing about thirty-six cubic inches of coarsely powdered peat charcoal. I have had this in continual action for three months; and although the charcoal has not been renewed, yet it does not show any sign of derangement or loss of power.

"All kinds of charcoal are not however, equally valuable for the purpose. Dr. Stenhouse found that wood charcoal and peat charcoal are the most effective. Mr. Blythe's experiments at the Board of Health, and the inquiries made in my own laboratory by Mr. Fewrell, are to the same effect. The cause of this superiority is doubtless due to the great porosity of vegetable charcoal. Liebig states that the pores in a cubic inch of beech-wood charcoal must, at the lowest computation, be equal to the surface of one hundred square feet, and several other chemists have estimated it at more than double this amount. Hence the extraordinary physical power of wood charcoal in condensing gases and vapors within its pores; so that when it is exposed to an atmosphere containing the putrid products of decomposition, it absorbs and oxydizes them by a species of combustion that is as effectual as if they were passed through the ignited coals of a furnace.

"Now in making a practical application to these facts, it is manifest that we have in common wood charcoal a powerful means of destroying foul gases of sewers. How it is to be applied is fortunately a question of but little embarrassment, for let the sewers be ventilated as they may, either by open gratings in the street or by the rain-water pipes of the houses, or by pillars of the gas-lamps, or by tubes carried up at the landlord's expense from the drains of every house, or by especial shafts of the public street—in fact, let the gases go out of the sewers how they will and where they will, you have but to place a small box containing a few pennies' worth of charcoal in the course of a draft, and the purification of the air will be complete."

System of Sewers.—To procure the most efficient system of sewerage, by a well-connected system of sewers, and to determine their proper level, and the degree of declination of which they are capable, according to the situation and nature of the soil of the place, as well as to ascertain what are the best materials for their construction, and the diameters best adapted to give them proper powers of transmission, are questions which, although they must be investigated and determined by the civil engineer, are still of lively interest to the professional sanitarian. Thus, for instance, he will tell us that the very large sized sewers, such as the *Cloaca Maxima*, unless intended for trunk sewers running the entire length of the city, are not serviceable. Egg-shaped culverts of a moderate size, and, preferably still, circular pipes of small diameter, and perfectly smooth and glazed, are superior, by far, to the sewer with upright sides and flattened segmental invert. It would be difficult to estimate the great amount that might be saved not only by a judicious system of sewerage, but even by a proper form of sewers, unless from data such as those furnished some years ago by Mr. Williams in his examination before Commissioners of whom we have precedingly spoken. In the Westminster district of London, in forty miles of covered drains built during a period of ten years, a loss of a sum equal to 333,348 dollars was incurred by faulty construction. In the whole metropolis, which includes the city of London, Westminster, the Holborn and Finsbury districts, and the Tower Hamlets, also the Surrey and Kent portions, which include the borough of Southwark, it appears that, during a period of ten years, about 220 miles of sewers were built. The difference between the expense actually incurred in this work by the construction of upright sided sewers with man-holes, and that which would have been required by egg-shaped or arched sewers, with a flushing apparatus, was a quarter of a million of pounds sterling, or about one million and two hundred and fifty thousand dollars. There is much less friction and risk of detention of sewage when the conveying duct is egg-shaped or circular. Even the opening of gully-holes, or the introduction of a gully-neck in the crown of the arch to admit the surface-water of the street into the sewer, produces accumulations. The plan so common in London of forming the opening of private or house-drains at right angles to the sewers, and, to aggravate the difficulty, of having them to approach the culvert at an elevation of eighteen inches or two feet above the latter, combines both objections; that of flattened invert and the junction of two sewers at right angles to each other. When sewers meet at right angles, there is a diminution of velocity, and eddies are formed, as well as injurious accumulations of deposit above the point of meeting; the rectangular mode of junction of the sewers increasing the resistance more than 200 per cent. It is of great importance that the internal surface of the sewer should be perfectly smooth, and in order to retain this property, that it should be built of indestructible materials, in part for reasons already assigned, and also to prevent inequalities and cavities from being formed, and the risk of falling of the entire wall by its becoming a burrow for rats, which have a great partiality for public sewers. Of equal necessity is a suitable declination in the line of the sewer, from its upper end, or in the heart of the city, to its termination in a river, or in a reservoir for the purpose. Mr. Hosking, whose calculations were made on certain low situations in Westminster, assumes that a fall of two inches the hundred feet, with a good back-water from a river, at equal intervals, would be sufficient.

So imperfect was the public drainage, not many years ago, in even the best parts of London, as in Regent street and Portland place, that, according to the testimony of Mr. Guthrie, before the Health of Towns Commissioners, there was not, at the time he made his observations in those streets, one gully clean in twenty that were not greatly choked up, and this even during heavy falls of rain. An idea may be had of the little interest felt in a system of progressive sewerage, from the fact, that in some large towns of England, as Wigan, Rochdale, and Bolton, there was not, some years since, the slightest knowledge of the plans of the sewers already made. Neglect of this kind should serve as a warning to the municipal governments in the United States to avoid similar faults.

The escape of deleterious emanations from sewers is prevented by traps or valves at the opening in the upper part, and the termination of the other end under water; and, if the opening at this end is exposed at low tides, by closing it with a gate. In London, Liverpool, and Glasgow, and in Paris and Hamburg, as well as in Boston, New York, and Philadelphia, the mouths of the sewers are exposed at low tide, and constitute an offense to the nostrils, and a probable source of disease. Of the ventilation of sewers we shall speak after awhile. Unless there be an abundant supply of water for keeping the lower and branch drains free from obstruction and accumulation, they will prove a source of annoyance and disease. To give effect to these means, a general and systematic survey of the different levels of a town should be made, and a uniform plan of sewerage adopted. Much trouble, expense, and sickness will be saved in its subsequent history, if these measures be adopted in the beginning of every new town. The rise of such is common enough in our widely extended country, in which the direct wants and necessities of trade, and emulous speculation are continually urging its people to new schemes—the foundation of a second Tyre or Alexandria, of another Persepolis, or Carthage, or Rome. As a general rule, each house-drain at least ought to be provided with a trap or valve to prevent the escape of emanations from the drain into the house. Especially is this necessary where the supply of water is not enough to keep the drain clean. Mr. Simpson, advocate of Edinburgh, urges strongly the advantage of a separation of sewers proper from surface-drains; the first holding sewerage proper, the second giving passage to rain and melted snow. He recommends the entire abandonment of *built* sewers, and the substitution of close pipes or tubes in their room.

The entire separation of sewerage from rain-fall is strenuously urged by Mr. F. O. Ward, in a letter to William Cuningham, Esq., Member of Parliament, in relation to the purification of the river Thames. Mr. Ward's cardinal proposition is, "that *the whole of the rain-fall* is due to the river, the whole of the sewage to the soil." And again, "that just as on the one hand, the sewage proper should be carefully diverted *from* the Thames, just so, on the other hand, should the rain-fall be directed *to* the Thames, to aid its scour—which suffers from every drop withdrawn. To divert a rain-brook is to mutilate a river." Both sewage and rain-falls are rendered useless by admixture.

The proportions of the two, apart from economical considerations connected with the disposal and utilization of sewage, forbid recourse to the same system of conduits for their conveyance. The average weight of the residuum (excluding moisture) yielded to the sewage by each man, woman, and child in London, is about two ounces *per diem*, and by the entire population, 139 tons in this period.* This is an insignificant quantity, if delivered as fast as produced. "But instead of taking measures to secure to London this regular decimal evacuation, we keep, on the most moderate estimate, at least twelve months' *excreta* constantly stagnating under ground, as deposit in the cess-pools and sewers. The mass of putridity thus constantly retained in subterranean London actually equals one day's evacuation of the whole population of Europe and Asia, numbering eight hundred millions."

The rain-fall on the London drainages, Mr. Ward thinks, may yield to the sewage some eighty or ninety millions of tons annually—a total about equivalent to the annual total of sewage. Were the fall of rain equally distributed throughout the year, it could, like the sewage, be easily disposed of.

* Dr. Letheby, as will have been seen in a preceding page, estimates the dry solid excreta of each inhabitant of the metropolis, to amount to from 2 to 2½ ounces, and the entire amount of solid matter contained in the sewage of one day, to be about 152.60 tons.

But so far from this being the case, the whole of the rain-falls on one hundred and fifty-two days of the year, and of the annual twenty-four inches, sixteen fall on forty-four days—or two thirds of the rain in about one eighth of the days. The disproportion between sewage and rain-fall is such, that, in one day in twelve, the former is to the latter as one to four and three quarters; in ten days in the year, as one to nine and a half; and on some few occasions, annually it is as one to nineteen, and upwards. Nor is the rain-fall assigned to each rain-day diffused over twenty-four hours of time; so that, for example, seven millions of tons of rain, equal to more than a month's sewage, sometimes fall on London in a single hour. "The mixed streams of rain-fall and sewage, liable to be thus suddenly swollen, exceed the capacity of any tunnels that can be built for their diversion from the river, and would overflow in any mechanism at our disposal for their distribution upon the soil."

Let us, with Mr. Ward, consider the effect of a sudden rainstorm falling on London, and pouring through the overcharged subterranean receptacles in the shape of sewers partially banked up with the accumulated sewage. Suppose it were to sweep into the river nine or ten days' accumulation of filth; this would be enough to discolor the tidal river, and in hot weather render its waters putrescent for several days. The money-loss on every such occasion would be, in ammonia only, without reckoning phosphorus, nearly sixteen thousand pounds sterling—$80,000.

Up to the point of meeting of the two streamlets, the one of the rain from roof and area, and the other of the sewage, from closet and sink, we are free to apply each of them to its proper use. "We can send the unpolluted rain-fall to scour the river, and the undiluted sewage to fertilize the land. But directly this junction-point is passed, directly the rivulet of cistern-water, rich with its freight of ammonia and phosphorus, meets and mingles with the casual rain-fall, the two waters become, as we have seen, a worthless, unmanageable mixture, equally unfit for agricultural and urban use. Not only do they cease to be our property, and pass beyond the control of art, but they revert to the domain of nature, spoiled even for her simple service. For this error we are punished by pestilence."

Mr. Ward speaks in terms of gratification at his having, with his friends, succeeded in establishing the tubular drainage of houses and streets, after a ten years' struggle with the engineers. The tubular sewers "are now working successfully by hundreds of miles, not only in provincial towns, but in the metropolis itself." The writer is confident "that this tubular purification of the Thames, will ultimately supersede the monstrous tunnel process, which, if adopted, would cost us many millions, and turn out a gigantic failure after all."

Dr. Huxley proposes to combine the embankment of the Thames on both sides, throughout the metropolis, with the formation of main sewer canals, the contents of which shall be subject to a tidal flushing towards the mouth of the river twice daily from flood to two thirds ebb. The fall in the canals should be only that of the river itself. At certain intervals, the canals would leave the river edge (the embankments to cease), and take a subterranean course by tunnels—five in number, and in length twenty miles on the north side, and three in number, and seventeen miles in length on the south side of the river. By means of the upper divergings from the river, the port of London would be left untouched, while the lower tunnels would obviate sharp bends in the river, which would offer obstacles if followed in the course of the canals.

The depth of the canals should be three feet below the lowest ebb of the stream; their height, four feet below the soil and pavement of the embankment. Taking the rise of the Thames at London Bridge at twenty feet, the canals would thus be twenty-five feet in depth, and the top of the embankment six feet above high water. The breadth of the canals might be determined according to the area required—say twenty feet, which would give a sectional area of five hundred square feet. All London surface-water, as well as sewage, should be allowed to enter the canals, both as an assistance to the movements of their contents, and a means of frequently lessening the amount of the river-water abstracted from the canals for the purposes of navigation.

If the saving of the sewage for the purposes of agriculture be a settled question, the required accessibility might be obtained at those points on the canals where it is proposed to make them open to the air (Rainham Creek, Gray's Thurrock, and Plumstead Marshes).

"Greatness of the cost is," Dr. Huxley thinks, "about the last consideration which ought to deter from any scheme embracing the power really to do the work. If five millions sterling were required and spent, five per cent thereon would not exceed two shillings per head *per annum* on the population of London."*

The editor of the *Sanitary Review*, Dr. Benjamin W. Richardson, in some remarks and suggestions on this subject (No. xiv.), while noticing the exaggerations respecting the existing evil, admits the necessity of cleansing the Thames, and that such arrangements should be made as shall at once lead to the constant and ready removal of the sewage with which the water is loaded. "Among the temporary plans for relieving the river of its dirty burden, the one most likely to answer the purpose for the present, and it may be for the future, consists in adopting for the direct removal of sewage, a system resembling the present water-conveyance system. A series of pipes laid down on the river-side to receive the sewage flow, and convey it towards the sea from the city,

* *Sanitary Review*, No. xiii.

would at once meet the emergency," as in the plan proposed by Mr. Austin, and in that as described, on a grand scale, by Dr. Huxley, just now placed before our readers.

"There is yet," writes Dr. Richardson, "another idea which has occurred to us, and which deserves at least as much consideration as the majority of the schemes which have been brought before the public. This idea suggests that floating reservoirs might be constructed for the reception of the sewer flow. We see no reason why the contents of a sewer might not be intercepted by a floating reservoir, through which the water part of the sewage might filter, and which, when charged with the solid and valuable sewage matter, might be lugged away for its contents, to be disembarked elsewhere, and disposed of for agricultural purposes. We doubt not, that with this arrangement rendered practicable, all the cost of sewage removal would be undertaken by private enterprise. The lading of sewage vessels with valuable cargoes, indeed introduces merely a new business for the river sailor."

In London, as we learn from the instructive "Report on the Results of Examinations made in relation to Sewerage in several European cities," by E. S. Chesbrough, Chief Engineer of the Board of Sewerage Commissioners, Chicago, there were, in a grand total of 934 miles of covered and 400 of open sewers, 126 of pipes, in 1855. The first pipe sewer was laid in 1848. The greatest length of any one is two and a half miles. Mr. Haywood, Engineer of the city of London, has always laid circular pipes; none smaller than nine inches, nor larger than fifteen inches diameter; the joints are put together sometimes with puddled clay, sometimes with cement.

The return of reflux odors, one of the greatest objections to house-drains, is prevented by three modes pointed out by Mr. Simpson: "First, the water pan *in* and the sigmatic curve under the water-closet and sink; next, another sigmatic curve, if the descent will make it safe, where the pipe joins the main street-drain; and thirdly, a delicately hung flap valve of galvanized iron at the extreme end of the tube, where it discharges into the main drain. The valve will always be shut, except when opened by a flow from the house." In the severe winters of our climate, obstructions to the easy working of these contrivances will not unfrequently occur, owing to the water freezing in the supply-pipe. For his sewers, Mr. S. rightly asserts that water in unstinted proportion is indispensable, but especially for a system of tubular sewers, which cannot be cleansed by any other method.

For drains, earthenware pipes, glazed, are preferable to brick conduits, which sometimes allow of exudation of their contents. The size of a pipe for a drain will depend on the number of houses. In one instance, in London, an 18-inch drain was carried 400 feet at the back of forty houses, where there was a good supply of water, and it was kept clean.

Robert L. Viele, Esq., Civil and Topographical Engineer, in a statement in the Senate Committee Report, expresses unhesitatingly his opinion, that one of the chief causes of mortality of the city of New York, "is to be found in the defective drainage of certain districts of the city, and furthermore, that this is an evil which is increasing as the city extends itself towards the northern portion of the island, and that the main elements by which this evil is increased, are the so-called city improvements, or grading of streets or avenues which are now being carried forward."

Mr. Viele then describes the intricate topography of the island of New York: "Abrupt ledges of rock, deep and narrow valleys, sudden upheavals and contortions of the geographical formations," with a surface varying in elevation from 5 to 150 feet above high-water mark. "Winding along this varied surface in every direction, are the original drainage streams, one of them of such an extent that it was formerly used for mill purposes." No attention having been paid to the original topography of the island, in the arrangement of streets and avenues, deep ditch excavations and high embankments have been made, so that these latter cross the old valleys of drainage, and become so many drains for the collection of water all over the island, which in summer are converted into "stagnant pools, breeding pestilence and disease." The earth dumped in to absorb the water, when it is desired to *improve* these lots, soon becomes saturated, and forms a sort of sponge through which the water ascends, and continues to be a permanent source of humid and noxious exhalations. No system of sewerage in which the sewers are only ten or twelve feet below the *grade* of the streets, can remedy this evil, when in some instances the underground streams are forty feet below the grade of the streets, "being thirty feet between the bottom of the sewer and the water of drainage." Melancholy evidence of the evils arising from habitation of a made soil, thus improperly drained, is afforded in the sacrifice of lives among the wretched victims sent to the present "Halls of Justice," or the "Tombs," as they are appropriately called, which are built on the site of the old Collect Pond, seventy feet deep—it was here that Fitch launched his first steamboat. The pond was connected with the Hudson River, by a stream running through what is now Centre and Canal streets; in this section of the city it is impossible to have dry cellars.

In giving farther currency to Mr. Viele's statement of the actual impediments to a complete system of drainage of the city of New York, and of his remedy, which we subjoin, our design is, as in the cases of hygienic deficiencies in other cities, not merely to incite to a reform in them, but also to furnish warning to new cities, or those in embryo, against the commission of similar mistakes and omissions in their incipient plans for civic improvement. Mr. Viele describes his remedial measures as follows:

"The remedy to be applied in the lower part of the city is

to widen the narrow streets, and to raise the grade where the streets pass through the original depression of the surface. Narrow streets, under any circumstances, are a curse to a city. They are too generally the abodes of vice and crime. In them an ordinary sickness spreads into a pestilence, and a fire into a conflagration. They are always filthy in summer, and frequently blocked up with snow in winter. They are not fit for business purposes, for they stifle commerce; nor for residences, for they breed disease. Wide streets, on the contrary, are more healthful and cheerful for residences, and more useful and valuable for business purposes. There is less danger from fire, as the flames cannot spread across the street. They are cleaner in summer, and are never impassable in winter. By constructing lateral drains along the slope of the depressions in the lower part of the city, and connecting them with the sewers, they will intercept the water in its descent, and prevent its accumulation in the original basins; and then raising the grade as is proposed in the accompanying profile of Worth street, at the same time widening the streets and perhaps discontinuing some of the short and insignificant streets in the 6th Ward, the health of the city will be improved one hundred per cent. So far as regards the upper part of the city, it is absolutely necessary that some system should be adopted for the free flow of water along the channels of the original drainage stream. This can be done by building more substantial culverts beneath the streets, and by the construction of permanent drains, so built as to admit of the percolation of water through the interstices of the covering. These drains should be excavated to a firm substratum, and every property owner should be compelled to construct, of a uniform character, that portion of each drain which may pass through his property."

Disposal of Sewage.—The subject of the application of sewage for agricultural purposes has been freely discussed of late years, especially in connection with its deodorization, and subsequently the free and more general use of it than could be obtained in its unaltered and offensive state. The practice of the Chinese, the most economical cultivators of the soil, is quoted at the same time, and their practice of uniting clay with fecal collections, and selling the compound for manure, referred to. Objections have been made to the deodorizing of sewage by chemical agents, on the ground of their neutralizing the ammonia, and destroying one of the most active of the exciters to vegetable growth. It has been computed, that if the whole drainage of London could be employed for manurial purposes at a sufficient distance from the city, the annual increase in the value of the land to which it would be applied, would exceed half a million of pounds sterling, or about two millions five hundred thousand dollars. An estimate by Mr. Smith, a distinguished agriculturist, places this question in a strong light. It rates the annual average value of the excreta of each individual at five dollars; so that, taking the whole population of Great Britain and Ireland at twenty-eight millions, we are positively, says this writer, *throwing away* every year that which is equivalent to *twenty-eight millions sterling*, or 140 millions of dollars. The actual salable value of the excreta in Belgium is thirty-seven shillings, and at this rate, continues the English writer just named, we may be said to be depositing the worth of fifty-one millions sterling in the ocean that washes our shores.

According to Dr. Lyon Playfair, a pound of urine is capable of increasing the production of grain by an equal weight; so that even allowing for some exaggeration in this estimate, the human urine wasted in the British kingdom would serve to produce more than all the grain required for the consumption of their entire population, besides affording through its fertilizing influence on lands at present imperfectly tilled, or not tilled at all, a source of employment to a superabundant laboring population.

Mr. Campbell, in an address on the utilization of sewage, says: "The chief element of the manurial value of town sewage is the excremental material, and this, in the instance of London, with a population of 2,600,000, amounts annually to 53,393 tons of dry solid,* which, as I have already shown, contains ingredients which give it a value of fifteen pounds sterling ($75) per ton, at least.

The quantity of ammonia which this contains,
or is capable of producing, is .... 11,440 tons.
The phosphoric acid, ... 1,839 "
And the potash, &c., ... 1,331 "

These three items make up a money value of about 836,834 pounds sterling, equal to 4,184,170 dollars.

The number of methods that have been proposed for obtaining manure from town sewage may be considered, Mr. Campbell thinks, under three heads.

1. Filtration through various media, and after the addition of chemical substances.

2. Precipitation by means of various re-agents.

3. Irrigation.

Reviewing the three modes here named, Mr. Campbell inclines to that by irrigation, and concludes, that by no process of chemistry hitherto known, can a highly valuable solid material be procured from town sewage alone.

Mr. Ward, in his letter to Mr. Cunningham, of which we have already made large use (p. 509), says on the present theme: "In the first place I would remind you, that to throw away the ammonia and the phosphorus of the London sewage, is virtually to throw away bread. Town sewage, which many engineers look upon as refuse to be discharged, I regard as property to be administered. The proper outfall for the London sewage is not this or that point of the river or of the sea,

* There must be some mistake in this estimate, which is not made more than a third of that made by Dr. Letheby.

but a suitable tract of land growing exhausting crops. "Fifty farms of a thousand acres each might be raised in value at least ten pounds per acre *per annum*, equivalent to five per cent. to ten millions of capital. This ought not to be thrown into the sea."

VENTILATION.—Two great requisites for the healthy existence of human beings, are due supplies of pure air and of pure water. Without these, the most abundant food and all the appliances furnished by science and art will be of little avail; and yet, by a singular inconsistency in human conduct, there would seem to be a fixed determination on the part of the majority of mankind to deprive themselves of these essential elements of health. Air, in an especial manner, is shut out from habitations by all kinds of contrivances, or, when allowed ingress, it is deteriorated by admixture with emanations from decayed organic matter, or from living bodies brought together in large numbers, to meet the wants of what is called civilization.

The atmosphere by which we are surrounded and from which, by means of respiration, our bodies derive the oxygen, or vital element of the air—that necessary for the support of life—is at the same time the great reservoir into which flow all the exhalations from the bodies of men and animals, and those resulting from the animal and vegetable decay which takes place on the surface of the soil. If not carried into space in the upper air by winds, tbey would prove a destructive poison to all the people congregated in cities and towns. The process by which those exhalations are removed is ventilation; and the more complete it is, the healthier are the inhabitants; as, on the other hand, its imperfection and neglect are productive of diseases of the worst kind. Streets are so many channels for conveying the requisite air to the inhabitants of the houses on either side of them;

and the wider and more numerous are these channels, the more completely is their object, in this respect, attained. Proportions ought to be preserved between the breadth of a street and the height of the houses in it. If the latter be very high, and the former narrow, both the air and sun are prevented from reaching the street, and lower portion of the houses. Still greater detriment, in this respect, is experienced by the occupants of narrow alleys and small courts, in which unfortunately the crowd of inhabitants is greatest, and the supply of fresh air and suitable ventilation the least. Every sanitary investigation, down to the last made in New York, goes to show the magnitude of the injury done to the public health by this last-mentioned state of things. The ills thence resulting are on the increase, since they follow, too generally, in certain but not well-defined proportions, the growth of the cities themselves. No excuse, therefore, will be offered for dwelling on this subject, first by presenting the darker and repulsive features, and then under its remedial and preventive aspect.

Few pause, says Dr. D. B. Reid, to consider the necessary consequence of 20 respirations per minute, 1200 per hour, or 28,800 in a single day and night for every adult human being, and of his abstracting, during this period of twenty-four hours, from the atmospheric magazine, his portion of air, amounting to fifty-seven hogsheads, of which he retains vital oxygen to the amount of about twenty pounds, that enters into his blood, and there serves to maintain the activity of all the functions of life, corporeal as well as mental. It has been estimated that about one fourth of all the air drawn into the lungs by inspiration is altered in these organs, and is no longer fitted for respiration. The alteration consists, first, in the abstraction of the vitalizing element of oxygen; and secondly, in the addition of the deleterious and poisonous gas—carbonic acid—which, together with volatilized animal matter, is given out by expiration, and passes into the outer and common atmosphere. But if, instead of a free inhalation of pure atmospheric air, there takes place that of a noxious or impure air, from which the exhaled carbonic acid has not been carried away, two results ensue: first, the individual fails to receive his proper proportion of oxygen, while he suffers from the inhalation of the noxious carbonic acid gas; and secondly, the lungs are unable to eliminate from the blood with their usual freedom the noxious products, including this very carbonic acid, or its base, carbon, the retention of which, together with the animal matter (previously mentioned) in the system, is productive of serious disorder in itself, and predisposes to the attacks of current diseases. This abnormal condition of things will continue, with aggravation, on to a fatal termination, if the same air be breathed over and over again, without its being displaced by a purer air; that is, without ventilation being carried on. Bad ventilation, as well said by Dr. Reid, is also injurious to the mind as to the body; and, where it is utterly neglected, not only produces headache and apoplexy, but, conjoined with other circumstances, is prone to favor that depression which leads at times to low spirits, and even to suicide.

Defective Ventilation—Crowded Streets and Habitations.—Taking into account the physiological data just mentioned in connection with the facts previously described, of the noxious effluvium of the gases resulting from the putrefaction of animal and vegetable matter, we find a ready explanation of the great amount of sickness and high death-rates among the crowded courts and cellar population in Liverpool, Birmingham, New York, and other cities. In Liverpool, in 1841, there were 2,398 courts containing 68,365 persons. In the parish of Birmingham, the older and more densely inhabited parts of the town, there were 2000 courts, containing 50,000 inhabitants. In Liverpool it was not enough, for outraging humanity and common-sense, that, gloomy and badly ventilated as the houses themselves were in the courts, there were found cellars under more than one half of them, or 1272 in number, occupied by 6290 persons. The whole number of cellars in Liverpool was 7892, containing a population of nearly 40,000 persons, or five persons on an average to each cellar. Aware, as we are, of the impossibility of a ventilation of these courts and cellars, and the continued deterioration of the air by exhalations from them and their inmates, we need not wonder at the bad eminence which that city, after the registration act had gone into full operation, unexpectedly acquired, on the score of disease, and the short average duration of life of its inhabitants, taking them in the aggregate. Reference has been made in a previous part of this report to the greater amount of sickness and mortality in the undrained than in the drained cellar districts of Liverpool. The concomitant evils attending this crowded population are tersely described by Dr. Reid, in speaking of the 8000 houses in Nottingham, built back to back and side to side, and with no other outlet than the street-door. "Suffice it to say, that in such quarters it is hardly possible that a family can preserve for any term of years, either decency, morals, or health." Worse, if possible, than the scenes exhibited in some English towns, is the condition of the poor in the chief cities of Scotland. Dr. Arnot, among other details, relates that in some of the wynds of Edinburgh and Glasgow, there were no sewers or drains, and the dung-heaps received all the filth which the swarm of wretched inhabitants could give: he learned that a considerable part of the rent of the houses was paid by the produce of the dung-heaps. The interior of these houses, and their inmates, corresponded with their exterior. "We saw half-starved wretches crowding together to be warm, and in one bed; although in the middle of the day, several women were imprisoned under a blanket, because as many others, who had on their backs all the articles of dress that belonged to the party, were then out of doors in the streets."

The pictures drawn some years back by Dr. J. H. Griscom, of the diseases and mortality caused by residence "in the damp, dark, and chilly cellars" of New York, and of "the degraded habits of life, the filth, the degenerate morals, the confined and crowded apartments, and insufficient food of those who live in more elevated soil, engendering a different train of diseases, failed to arrest the attention of the authorities. The evils have been allowed to go on increasing, until at last their alarming excess has led to official investigations, the results of which fully confirm all that Dr. Griscom, and other sanitarians on the spot, had previously proclaimed. They are embraced in a "Report of the Select Committee appointed to investigate the Health Department of the City of New York," which, together with a large amount of appended documents, in the shape of medical and other testimony, and tabular matter, was transmitted to the Legislature, February 3, 1859. A startling fact which tells in a few figures the deplorable state of the public health in the city of New York, is its gradual deterioration, with some interruptions and short rises, during the last forty-six years. Thus, we learn that in 1810, with a population of 96,713, the deaths were 1 in 46.6; whereas, in 1857, with a population of probably 700,000, the deaths were 1 in 27.15. The testimony of Dr. Griscom, in Committee, is full of instructive details, direct and comparative, on the subject of the causes of the increase of death-rates in New York. He shows that if the mortality of London bore the same ratio as that of New York to population, it would have been 92,784, in place of 56,786, which was its actual mortality. Dr. G. quoted from the Report of a Committee of the Association for Improving the Condition of the Laboring Classes in the City of New York, in which the dwellings in many parts of the city are thus characterized:

"Crazy old buildings; crowded rear tenements in filthy yards, dark, damp basements, leaky garrets, shops, out-houses, and stables, converted into dwellings, though scarcely fit to shelter brutes, are the habitation of thousands of our fellow-beings in this wealthy, Christian city." "In Oliver street, Fourth Ward, for example, is a miserable rear building, 16 feet by 30, two stories and garret, three rooms to each of the first and second floors, and four in the attic; in all, ten small apartments, which contain *fourteen families.* The entrance is through a narrow, dirty alley, and the yard and appendages of the filthiest kind." In Cherry street, is a "tenement-house," in two lots, extending back from the street about 150 feet, five stories above the basement, so arranged as to contain 120 families, or more than 500 persons. "But the most objectionable habitations in this district are the cellars, in some instances six feet under ground, which have to be bailed out after every rain-storm, and are so damp as to destroy health, so dark as to prevent industry, and so low that ventilation is impossible. Though utterly unavailable for every other use, they are rented, at rates which ought to procure comfortable dwellings, to persons who have become as debased in character, as the condition is degrading, in which they live." Many of the poor of the Sixth Ward "are in a condition incomparably worse than the hovel-dwellers, where father, mother, children, and swine live and lodge together." In the Eighth Ward, "Rotten Row," so unlike the fashionable locality in London thus called, "consists of eight houses on either side of the street, fronting each other, with as many more in the rear, containing, in all, about two hundred and fifty families, and not less than one thousand two hundred and fifty persons, in a space of about one hundred and eighty feet, by, perhaps, a depth of fifty feet on each side. The pestiferous stench and filth of these pent-up tenements exceed description. In one room, says a visitor, six people are living, with hens scratching about on the bed. Every corner of these buildings is occupied—cellars and garrets." The cellar population of New York is believed to be twenty-five thousand. What makes the case worse with the occupants of these tenements and cellars, is, the circumstance of many of them being emigrants from Europe, particularly from Ireland and Germany, who, during their voyage, had suffered from defective ventilation, in their being crowded between decks, and compelled to breathe much of their time a damp and impure air. Among the diseases arising from, or singularly multiplied and aggravated by, what Dr. Griscom terms "internal domiciliary causes," are Cholera Infantum, Diarrhœa, and Erysipelas, which have been increased in a high proportion since 1820.

Dr. Samuel Rotton, in his testimony before the Committee, repeating, in a summary manner, what had been said by Dr. Griscom, and, to a certain extent, also by Dr. McNulty, affirms the chief causes of the mortality in New York to arise from a great number of the inhabitants living "with the smallest amount of air that is necessary to keep life in them, and the smallest possible quantity of light with which they can possibly see and get along with; and these causes have been proven by Dr. Griscom to produce much greater mortality than bad food or bad clothing, because, the people who have lived in the same way, with the same food and clothing, in better localities, have been seventy-five *per centum* better with regard to mortality than those who lived in cellars and other dark, unventilated, and miserable places." During the cholera season of 1849, in New York, Dr. Rotton noted the fact of the great mortality from the disease among the occupants of cellars, and hence, it became his invariable practice to have such persons, when attacked, immediately removed. He does not know of a single case of recovery of those who were not removed. "The reason is obvious," continues Dr. R. "In many of them I was obliged to wade my way upon bricks, before I could stand upon the floors, for the water would cover my feet." In the same year, Dr. Rotton attended a great many patients who were attacked with Typhus or Ship Fever, and with results similar to those just noticed in regard to Cholera. All whom he could not remove from the cellars, died—whereas, those who were situated in well-ventilated places fared much better. He mentions the cases of two men lying sick with Typhus Fever, "in a back alley-way." His constant recommendation, at every visit, to admit fresh air, was as constantly disregarded, and on his return, each day, he found the windows again closed, the door closed, and a number of persons living in the same room with the sick. At last, Dr. Rotton, becoming exasperated, broke out every pane of glass in the upper portion of the windows. His patients gradually improved, and recovered. Dr. D. Meredith Reese, in his testimony before the Committee, lays down the proposition, that "The true criterion and best index of atmospheric impurity, in any city, or other locality, is manifested in young children, whose greater susceptibility to morbid causes, by reason of their greater delicacy of structure, renders them the earliest victims of atmospheric poisons. Hence the fearful aggregate of infant mortality in New York, which authentic statistics disclose, is at once the fruit and the proof of the contaminated air they breathe, in the wretched habitations of the poor, where confined and ill-ventilated apartments render healthy respiration impossible." Dr. Reese assigns other causes for infant mortality, which do not come under our present head, but which are suggestive of the importance and necessity of sanitary reform, not only in New York, but in most other cities. His views on the exceedingly interesting topic of infant mortality in large cities, have been embodied in a Report to the American Medical Association, which he offered as part of his testimony before the New York Committee.

The morbid effects of crowding and deficient ventilation are well illustrated by comparison with an opposite condition of things, as set forth by Dr. Richard S. Kissam. The comparison is of the state of health of two wards in New York, the most healthful and the least healthful. In the Sixth Ward there were twenty-five thousand inhabitants in 1856, having one thousand four hundred dwellings, and the deaths were one thousand and eighty-nine. In the Fifteenth Ward the population was twenty-four thousand and forty-six, who occupied two thousand four hundred and forty-five dwellings, and the deaths among whom were four hundred and thirty-six. The proportion of deaths in the Fifteenth Ward is one in fifty-five, and in the Sixth Ward one in twenty-three. The contrast, as set forth in the Report itself, between the Fifteenth and the First Wards in 1857, was still greater. The proportions were 1 in 69.68 in the former, and 1 in 21.96 in the latter. Dr. Kissam states the difference between New York and Philadelphia, on the score of public health, to be, that almost every family in the latter city has a tenement in itself; the members of it are well provided and comfortable. "The city, of course, has a larger number of houses in proportion than our own. It is very seldom that there is more than one family in a house; but here, as has been stated, there are twenty or thirty families in one house." To the question, "Then you regard ventilation as a great principle connected with the preservation of health?" Dr. Kissam replies: "Most assuredly, even in higher walks than among the poor. Our Academy of Medicine will sit, night after night, being poisoned, so that those who are sensitive on this point, invariably have a headache the next day. The Historical Rooms, the new building, is very badly ventilated. The subject of ventilation is one that seems to escape the attention of builders as well as of officers."

Examples of the connection of overcrowding with the development of Typhus, Scarlatina, and Cholera, are numerous. Some striking cases of this nature are recorded by Mr. Cox, in the *Sanitary Review*, April, 1858. In the limits of two streets, in the village of Bromley, fifty-three cases of fever occurred. The disease did not extend to the rest of the village, neither did it break out elsewhere within the district. The evident cause of this local fever, and its mortality, was the "awful" overcrowding. Each house consisted of four rooms, about twelve feet square. "An entire family lived and slept in each chamber. In one, Mr. Cox counted seven human beings, who occupied the same filthy couch—a father, mother, three adult daughters, and two younger children. In a second room, six persons slept, viz., a widow, her two grown-up daughters, an adult son, and two young children." It is unnecessary to say that the rooms were indescribably foul, fetid, close, and disgusting. "In the above instance," continues Mr. Cox, "we can have no hesitation in ascribing the concentration and severity of the fever-poison (if not indeed its actual development) to the vitiated atmosphere produced by the overcrowding." He made every inquiry, but was quite unable to trace the origin of the disease to any other sources. Dr. Duncan, of Liverpool, described, some years ago, a filthy, pent-up court, one of the thousands in that city, with an area of only one hundred and fifty square yards, occupied by one hundred and eighteen inhabitants, or about one and a quarter square yards to each. This average breathing room is only one half of what it ought to be at night. In this court, fifty cases of fever, or nearly one half the population, were attended by the Dispensary in a single year. Some of the most frightful ravages of Cholera on record were owing to the direct pulmonary poisoning by impure air and animal effluvium, accumulated for want of suitable ventilation. Examples of this nature have been furnished in all parts of the civilized world—in the East Indies, at Karrachee, among the troops, at Juggernaut, among the native population, also in the crowded and ill-ventilated barracks; in England, among the brickmakers at Southal, the hop-pickers at East Farleigh, the pauper children at Tooting, the lunatics in the Wakefield Asylum, the convicts at the Wakefield Old Prison, the inmates of the Millbank Penitentiary, and of the Taunton Work-house. At a time when no case of Cholera had occurred in the neighborhood of Tooting, and when, indeed, even Diarhœa was not at all prevalent in the village, three hundred of the inmates of the establishment were smitten with the secret pestilence, and of these no less than one hundred and eighty died. The girls, whose dormitories were the most overcrowded and the worst ventilated, suffered more severely than the boys. The essential cause of all this mortality was declared to be "the inordinate crowding of the establishment." The numbers crowded together into the dormitories were so great, that each boy had only one hundred and fifty cubic feet, and each girl one hundred and thirty-three cubic feet of air allowed for respiration, and some of the apartments were, at the same time, so faultily constructed—there being windows on one side only—that no effective ventilation could possibly be kept up.

How far this scant supply of the *pabulum vitæ* falls short of the requirements of health, may be inferred from the recommendation of the inspectors of prisons in England, some years ago, that every prisoner should have one thousand cubic feet of air, and from the estimates which have been made in other quarters, that health and strength cannot be maintained in a space of less than seven hundred to eight hundred cubic feet; and that to live and sleep in a space less than four hundred to five hundred cubic feet for each individual, is not compatible with safety to life, even where there is no extrinsic or superadded cause of atmospheric impurity. And let it not be supposed that even the first-named spaces would be sufficient in a hermetically-closed box or chamber, for life would become extinct long before the oxygen had been consumed.* In Philadelphia, we have had some sad reminders of the pernicious effects of overcrowding and want of ventilation in the mortality, and preceding horrors in the old Arch Street Prison, during the cholera season of 1832, and in the Blockley Almshouse in the epidemic of 1849. We may note also similar catastrophes in the Bucks County Poorhouse, and the Baltimore Almshouse. Although Philadelphia, Boston, and Baltimore compare advantageously with New York in their annual death-rates, yet they have also their dark spots, their bad districts, in which physical is associated with moral degradation and impurity, and Cholera claims its largest proportion of victims. Whatever effects may be attributed to bad or defective supply of food in the production of this disease, it has been said, with no doubt much truth, that the state of health, as well as the proclivity to disease, is influenced much more by the condition of the air that is breathed than of the food that is eaten. The foul and fetid atmosphere, continues the English writer,† of our Whitechapels, and Bermondseys—aided often by intemperance—has more to do with the haggard looks and earthy complexion of these denizens than even penury or want. Dr. Letheby, in visiting some of the rooms tenanted by poverty-stricken beings crowded together, found the atmosphere so close and unwholesome, and infected with that peculiar fainty and sickening smell so characteristic of the filthy haunts of poverty, that he endeavored to discover the special offending element. He ascertained that the contaminated and reduced air was not only deficient in due proportion of oxygen, but that it contained three times the usual amount of carbonic acid, besides a quantity of alkaline matter that stank abominably, doubtless the

* Brit. and For. Med.-Chir. Review, vol. vii., 1851.

† Ibid.

product of putrefaction of the various fetid and stagnant exhalations that are given off from the unclean body, and a pestilential scourge of disease, the consequence of heaping human beings into such contracted localities.

Observations have been made, and to such an extent as to justify the belief, that the intensity and mortality of Scarlet Fever are greatly increased by overcrowding. Mr. Cox, already quoted, describes an outbreak of this Fever with fearful and uncontrollable malignity in a dismal court at the back of Covent Garden, London. There were altogether nineteen cases in the three houses, whereof ten terminated fatally. Mr. Cox "can confidently attribute this fearful mortality to the overcrowding; as, although the disease prevailed extensively in the neighboring streets, it did not assume the same malignity of type, and yielded to remedial measures." Both Mr. Cox and a friend who accompanied him, and shared the professional duties with him on his visits to this forbidding spot, contracted the disease, and narrowly escaped with their lives. Measles have nearly double the mortality in the crowded north-western districts, that they have in comparatively thinly peopled south and south-east ones of England. Even though we must attribute a good deal to the ready transmission of contagious disease among a thickly planted population, we can hardly doubt, as suggested by Mr. Simon, that a general weakness of constitution, conjoined with defective sanitary arrangements, greatly aggravates the fatality of the contagious diseases in question.

Predilection of Cholera for Old Haunts of Disease.—Dr. Laycock, in his highly interesting report to the Health of Towns Commissioners, on the Epidemics of York, tells us, that the first steps of the plague which used to ravage that ancient city in the middle ages, down to the early part of the seventeenth century, seem to have been very similar to those of the cholera in 1831, marking the badly-drained districts by its course, as did the latter. "It is a singular coincidence," remarks Dr. Laycock, "that while the cholera commenced in the Hay-market, near the traditional spot of the plague under consideration (in 1604), and probably near to that of 1551, the first death from cholera took place also in the parish of St. Michael, Spurriengall, and on June 5th." It was in this parish, and on June 4th, 1604, that the first death from plague occurred. The first case that occurred in the town of Leith (Edinburgh), in 1848, took place in the same house, and within a very few feet of the same spot where the epidemic of 1832 commenced its course. On its re-appearance in the town of Pollockshaws, it snatched its first victim from the very same room and the very bed in which it had broken out in 1832. Its first appearance in Bermondsey was close to the same ditch in which the earlier fatal cases occurred in 1839. At Oxford, in 1839 as in 1832, the first case occurred in the county jail. This return to its former haunts has been observed in several other places, and the experience in foreign countries has been similar. At Groningen, in Holland, the disease in 1832 attacked, in the better part of the city, only two houses, and the epidemic broke out in these two identical houses on the visitation of 1848. But it was observed, that while in both epidemics, those of 1832 and 1848–9, the disease was localized in precisely the same districts, several of them have changed places in the relative degree in which they have suffered The earliest case of cholera in Chelsea (near London), in 1848, is said to have been in Whitehall Court, and there it continued to exist until the end of the epidemic in 1849. The first case in 1854 was in the same place, perhaps also in the same house, in both visitations. A very similar fact is presented by Augusta Court, in which the three earliest fatal cases of cholera, in Chelsea, occurred in February, 1832; and which being revisited in 1854, continued to furnish victims to the pestilence throughout the early duration of the outbreak. Kent and Mew streets, Southwark (on the south side of the Thames), which were severely visited at an early period of the last epidemic, were also among the first seats of cholera in 1832. Dr. Acland relates that, with one exception, every yard and every street in St. Thomas's parish, Oxford, which had been attacked by cholera in 1832 and 1849, was revisited in 1854.

It is evident, from these and many more analogous facts, that, although we are unable to explain all the conditions for the development of cholera, it is impossible for us to deny the great influence of locality on its production.

Public Lodging-Houses.—To speak of overcrowding is at once suggestive of public lodging-houses, long a recognized and prolific source of disease and vice. They are in all large cities the nightly resorts, not only of the migrating laborer and traveling artisan, but, also, of the lower mendicants, thieves, and prostitutes. It was no uncommon thing, as Dr. Duncan related, when writing on the sanitary state of Liverpool, for the keepers of lodging-houses, in that city, to cover the floor with straw, and to allow as many human beings as could manage to pack themselves together, to take up their quarters for the night, at the charge of a penny (a little over two cents) each. The havoc made by the cholera in the lodging-houses of Manchester was terrible. In some of them as many six or eight bodies were contained in a single room, which was crowded promiscuously with men, women, and children. Dr. Howard, after showing the lamentable extent to which they become hot-beds of febrile diseases of the most violent and fatal character, owing mainly to their filthy and unventilated condition, thus describes the morals of their frequenters, and their malign influence in this way on the young and inexperienced: "They serve as open receptacles of crime, vice, and profligacy, and as nurseries in which the young and yet uninitiated become familiar with every species of immorality. They are the haunts of the most depraved and abandoned characters, as well as the most miserable and suffering objects of the town (Manchester), and constitute one of the most influential causes of the physical and moral degradation of our laboring population." In Glasgow, where the same evils prevailed to an alarming degree, the lodging-houses have been subjected to regular municipal supervision and ordinance, and, as we are told, with excellent effects. Partial inquiries made in our large American cities, reveal a state of things approaching to the evils just pointed out as so common in those of Great Britain, and which call imperatively for the ameliorating and reforming influences introduced with success of late years in different parts of this kingdom. To these we shall soon advert.

General Want of Ventilation.—But the evil consequences of crowding and defective ventilation are not confined to the poor and the destitute. Wherever people are brought together for religious worship, for amusement or recreation, in the halls of legislation and of law, in school-rooms, hospitals almshouses, and prisons, the neglect of sanitary measures, and especially of ventilation, is the rule. Attention to this paramount means of preserving health is the exception. Nor are the mansions of the rich and tasteful exempt from the penalty of infraction of one of the chief if not the very first of the natural laws. This stricture is still more applicable to modern than to old houses.

In modern houses, the neglect of ventilation is extreme, as far as regards recourse to any other means of obtaining it than the windows of the rooms. All the fire-places, as they used to be called, are hermetically sealed by slabs of marble, and when the register of the flue, by which warm air is introduced, is closed, as at night, or when the room becomes too warm in the day, there is no aperture, either for the admission of fresh air from without, or for the escape of foul air from within. During the night, the windows and doors are closed, and the supply of air fitted for respiration becomes exhausted long before morning, especially if, as is so commonly the case, there be several persons sleeping in the same room. Headaches, restless slumbers, nervousness of various kinds, palpitations, oppressed breathing, and loss of appetite, are no unusual effects of defective ventilation in the houses of the wealthy, who, at the very time, may be commiserating the poor for their small and close apartments. It is indeed time that architects should wake up, and think of constructing houses in which the inmates can live without a continued infraction of the laws, by compliance with which alone they can enjoy health and serenity of mind. Benevolent individuals and societies have taken the state of the defective lodgings of the poor into consideration, and have set about, in some instances with entire success, the devising and execution of the needful remedies. Let us hope that the rich will, in due time, come in for a share of this well-directed philanthropy.

We hear much of applied science, but the community has yet to learn its direction towards a better system of either public or private hygiene. Both proprietors and builders of houses are, for the most part, quite innocent of the desired knowledge of this subject. Division of rooms for business or family wants in the interior, and decorations externally after some order, Greek or Gothic, or a barbarous blending of both, are the only things thought of in relation to modern structures. How the inmates are to procure an adequate and continued supply of fresh air, and how to get clear of that which is impure, are not even secondary matters: they are sometimes discussed as curious questions of philosophy, but seldom with a view to their direct bearing on health. Wearied, oppressed, and giddy, and with palpitating hearts and hurried breathing, how many, after leaving a church, have mistaken their really disturbed states of the physical man for those which result from the workings of the Spirit; and have retired to their homes, full of terrors for the state of their soul, when, in reality, they were suffering from a disorder of their corporeal functions, induced by the impure and half-poisoned blood circulating through their veins? We are familiar with the "blue Monday" of dissipated and drunken workmen and laborers, who pay the penalty of a recognized gross infraction of natural laws on the preceding Sunday, but we are not often aware of the well-defined "blue Monday," as exhibited in feelings of languor, depression of spirits, and unevenness of temper in those who have sinned against these same natural laws, albeit in a different manner, by their three goings to church, including an evening service on the Sabbath, and breathing all the while an impure air. Dr. D. B. Reid, who visited numerous churches in hot weather, to observe the effects of bad air on the congregations, gives the result in a very graphic sketch, which we regret not having room to insert. We would refer to his work, entitled *Illustrations of the Theory and Practice of Ventilation, with remarks on Warm Air, Exclusive Lighting, and the Communication of Sound*, for much valuable information on the entire subject embraced in our present notice.

The same author has favored the public with a more recent treatise on *Ventilation in American Dwellings*, with a series of illustrative diagrams; and to this eminently practical work, Dr. Elisha Harris has contributed an *Introductory Outline of the Progress of Improvement in Ventilation.* The volume is replete with instruction on a most interesting, we might say vital topic.

Dr. E. Harris, after stating "the imperative necessity of giving prompt and efficient attention to the removable sources of danger and disease which exist in our communities," presents the subject in a very lucid manner in the shape of the following propositions:

"*First.* We would refer to the fact that more than one half the entire population of the city of New York reside in crowded tenement-houses, and that there is no statute or municipal law regulating the construction, ventilation, or the space allowed to specified numbers of residents therein. Hence crowding such structures to their utmost capacity has become the rule rather than the exception. And it may here be stated, that our city has an underground or cellar population of more than twenty-five thousand persons.

"In the 17th Ward alone, there are 1257 tenement-houses, having 20,917 rooms, which are occupied by 10,123 families, embracing a total number of 51,172 persons; thus giving an average of about four persons to each suit of two apartments, one only of which is usually occupied as a dormitory, and that one often a dark, close room, of a capacity only of from 500 to 800 cubic feet. Now, in a close apartment of only 600 cubic feet, a single person cannot spend six consecutive hours, in air of ordinary temperature, without impairment to health.

"Dr. Reid's estimate of ten cubic feet of pure air per minute, for the respiration of an adult person, is certainly quite low enough for an average of comfort and safety, and with such an allowance, the air in such an apartment would become too much vitiated for healthy respiration at the expiration of sixty minutes or one hour; and allowing that the air is partially replenished during that brief period, the atmosphere would be decidedly unwholesome at the expiration of two or three hours. Or, taking the lowest estimate within the limits of safety, as given by Dr. Neill Arnott, viz., about three cubic feet per minute, such an apartment could not be considered a healthy sleeping-room for a single person. much less a safe dormitory for a whole family.

'In some of the lower wards of the city, the tenement-houses are much more densely crowded than in those just mentioned. In one of them, containing from 120 to 150 families of three to ten persons each, there are but about forty feet of frontage and sunlight. In two of the smallest of those apartments, eight cases of malignant typhus have been seen at one time. And at the last visitation of cholera, the first cases of that malady occurred in that pent-up and overcrowded locality.

"*Second*, Small-pox, typhus fever, and every other pestilence find a genial and prolific soil in such crowded, unventilated structures as the habitations of the poor in our city, and from them the germs of fatal diseases are continually conveyed to the dwellings of the more favored classes.

"*Third*, The fashionable and gregarious custom of crowding our hotels and boarding-houses is becoming a hazardous practice, unless more attention is given to the hygienic condition and wants of such establishments—very few of which have hitherto been provided with any thing like systematic and efficient ventilation, or perfect drainage. The recent fearful endemic at the National Hotel, in the city of Washington, should teach an important practical lesson on this subject.

"*Fourth*, The drainage or sewerage, and the necessary measures for securing general cleanliness and a pure atmosphere, are not yet suitably provided for by law.

"*Fifth*, Architecture, in its applications to private residences as well as to public edifices, has not yet had primary or suitable reference to man's hygienic interests. Adaptations for a sufficient supply of pure air and sunlight have been sacrificed to architectural effect on the one hand, and to a mistaken economy on the other.

"The vital importance of a correct understanding and estimation of such considerations as the foregoing, must be manifest to all who intelligently investigate such subjects; and to the political economist, the merchant, and the moralist, these topics are invested with relations quite as interesting as those that lead the physician and the philanthropist to study them."

Dr. Reid was one of the Commissioners appointed by Queen Victoria for inquiry into the state of large towns and populous districts; and his opinions are founded on large experience

In Schools.—The greatest sufferers from the general ignorance of elementary physiology and hygiene among architects, controllers and teachers, are children in schools, both public and private; the latter just now probably the more punished of the two. We need not repeat from the report of the Commissioners just mentioned, the distressing particulars of the wretched state of the cottage schools in the different parts of England, nor of the dame and public schools of Liverpool and Manchester some years ago. Abundant matter for comment and stricture is offered to observation in the schools of the United States. The fate of the school children of poor or improvident parents, who reside in narrow streets, courts, or alleys, is peculiarly hard; for, after suffering from partial suffocation during the night and a part of the day in their own wretched homes, they are subjected to a similar, if not more injurious process in their school-rooms, into which they may be said to be entrapped, and thus cruelly treated under the show of kindness and regard for their welfare.

Of all the various edifices in which a number of persons are gathered together, and for whose protection and benefit an efficient system of ventilation is needful, none are of such paramount importance as school-houses, and none have been so generally, and we might add so cruelly neglected. The children who sit in them for many hours daily, require, above all other members of the community, a continued supply of fresh air for their healthy growth, and to allow of their tender brains being tasked without detriment and continual danger to their intellects, and a depression of spirits and languor so opposed to their instinctive feelings and tendencies. The originally indolent boy becomes at school a hater of lessons and books, associating as he does with it all that is wearisome and dull; while the boy desirous to learn, and emulous of distinction, becomes exhausted by his brain-work, and his nervous system acquires a morbid sensibility which remains with him during all his after-life. The unrenewed air of a school-room soon becomes charged with the noxious exhalations both from the lungs and the skin. The latter organ, in a vast majority of the poorer children, and in not a few of the wealthier class, becomes, for want of due attention, almost coated with perspirable and other matters, and is a source of continual poisoning of the air of an ill-ventilated room. The architectural arrangement of nearly all the schools in England, as far as they were examined some years ago, was, with few exceptions, deplorably defective, especially where the scholars slept in the building. Among many instances of the same kind, we may state that, in Manchester, the blue-coat boys suffered from scurvy, which was removed in a great measure by an amended diet, and by ventilation of the dormitories after a fixed method. But it is not necessary to look abroad to find a general neglect of school hygiene, evidenced even in what all call first-class seminaries, as well as in those of less pretension and with humbler inmates.

In Hospitals.—All medical men must be aware, at the present time, how much the mortality is increased in hospitals and asylums of every kind by a confined air, rendered noxious by want of ventilation. The greatest skill on the part of the professional corps, the most attentive administration of well-selected medicines by intelligent and humane nurses, are nullified by the inmates of a hospital breathing an air not continually renewed, and which, if allowed to remain stationary, even for a very short period, becomes charged with emanations, gaseous and animal, of the most deleterious kind. It is not too strong language to say, that a renewal of the air in hospitals, which implies adequate ventilation, is a question of life or death: every hospital in which the atmospheric air remains vitiated, so far from being a benefit to the poorer classes, becomes a public calamity. Better that its inmates should remain in their own wretched tenements, deprived of all medical attendance, than to be subjected to the concentrated poison of the large wards of a hospital. Many years ago, during a season of epidemic visitation of small-pox in Philadelphia, it was found that the mortality from this disease was greater among the inmates of the hospital at Bush Hill, of which your reporter was at the time the chief medical attendant, than among the sick in the city, many of them living in confined courts and dirty alleys, who came under his care as dispensary patients. As illustrative of the contrasted effects of crowding and bad ventilation on the one hand, and of improved ventilation on the other, reference may be made to the Lying-in Hospital, Dublin, in which there died 2,944 children out of 7,650; but after ventilation, the deaths, in the same period of time, and in a like number of children, amounted only to 279. Tho quantity and poisonous nature of the exhalations continually given out in the wards of a hospital occupied by the sick, are strikingly shown by Montfalcon and Polinière in a treatise on the Health of Great Cities,* when speaking of the *Hotel Dieu*, the great hospital at Lyons. The large fever wards of this building represent a cross, at the centre of which is a vestibule surmounted by a dome and a cupola; in it is placed an altar of marble, over which is a smaller dome. From the wards thus communicating with the vestibule, the impure air and exhalations escape into the dome and cupola, which act as so many funnels, and thence through suitable openings they find exit into the outer air. The

* Traité de la Salubrité dans les Grandes Villes, suivie de l'Hygiene de Lyon.

amount of mephitic air accumulated in the dome and cupola, and afterwards expelled, is incredible, as no one could form the least idea of it when visiting the wards and breathing an air exempt from all bad smell in them. But if workmen at this very time ascend to the cupola, especially near its top, they will suffer so much from the close and foul air which has risen from below, as to be unable to continue their work, at the longest, for more than half an hour. Sometimes even after half an hour's delay in this infectious medium, they come away pale and oppressed, and so disordered that sometimes they sink down in a state of syncope. Many workmen are obliged to succeed one another, to perform the work of a single man.

In Work-shops and Factories.—The work-shops of persons engaged in various mechanical employments are for the most part exceedingly deficient on the score of ventilation, and their inmates in consequence encounter much suffering and disease. Dr. Southwood Smith relates many distressing details of this nature, which came under his own observation. There was a room in London, sixteen or eighteen yards long, and seven or eight yards wide, in which eighty working tailors sat, and so closely to each other, as to be nearly knee to knee; one witness told of his having known young men, tailors from the country, faint away in the shop from the excessive heat and closeness. It was of frequent occurrence in such work-shops, that suits of clothes of a light color were spoiled from the perspiration of the hand, and the dust and flue which arose during the work. In winter, these places are still more unhealthy, as the heat from the candles—it may now be said gas—and the closeness are much greater. The entrance of fresh air through an open window is objected to by those nearest to it on account of the draught, and generally they prevail in keeping out the cold—that is, the fresh air. The effects of continued exposure to this impure and deleterious air, were to drive away many before their labors were over, and to take away the appetite of those unaccustomed to the place. "The natural effect of the depression," continues the witness before the Commissioners, "was that we had recourse to drink as a stimulant; gin being taken instead of food. I should say the greater part of the habit of drinking was produced by the state of the place of work, because when men work by themselves, or only two or three together, in cooler and less close places, there is scarcely any drinking between them."

Seamstresses, &c.—What has been said of the journeymen tailors, applies with too much force to the individuals of the other sex, who work in milliner and dressmaker shops, with the additional aggravation of their being sometimes kept up late at night to finish the dress promised by the employer for the next day. Even when working alone in their small and close rooms, from morn to night, in a half-bent posture, they are objects of deserved pity, as victims to the sin of a neglect of hygiene.

Printing Offices, in which germinate so many young Franklins, do not exhibit, if we may judge from the indifference of those who work within them, the shrewdness of their professed model, in either devising or availing themselves of known measures for the promotion of health, foremost of which is attention to the respiratory function. If it be true, as alleged, that pressmen are less liable than compositors to pulmonary consumption, we have additional confirmation of the fact, pointed out by Dr. Guy, of the greater frequency of this disease among those who are habitually exposed to a close and impure air, and especially if, at the same time, they are deprived of all exercise. The saving nature of this last is evinced under the circumstances just stated.

Nautical hygiene shows that outbreaks of cholera have occurred aboard ship from defective ventilation.

Pulmonary Diseases from Defective Ventilation.—It has been observed that, as a general rule, the frequency of pulmonary diseases in England is greater among the males than among the females, in the proportion of 100 to 94—as regards the country generally; but that in particular districts and towns, the greatest death-rates from these causes are on the side of the females. The difference is attributable to the confinement in factories or in shops, and even in their own houses, of this part of the population, while engaged in making textile or other fabrics. In three of the registration disricts in which this difference prevails, a good proportion of the adult females are engaged in industrial manufacturing pursuits—these being chiefly conducted at their own homes. Exceptions, not yet explained, occur in this matter in some counties in England. We are, after all, safe in adopting the opinion expressed by Mr. Simon, namely: "In proportion as the male and female populations are severally attracted to indoor branches of industry, in such proportion, other things being equal, their respective death-rates by phthisis are increased." In the lace-making districts, the female death-loss seems always to exceed the male. "The pulmonary death-rate is usually excessive in towns where both males and females are largely employed in the manufacture of textile fabrics; but the difference in the mortality of the sexes is rarely great." So in Manchester, which, as one of the cotton manufacturing districts, has a high pulmonary mortality, the difference in the death-rates of males and females is slight; both being largely engaged in the industrial occupations of the place. In comparing this state of things with what occurs in Liverpool, we find that city, with a higher mortality still, does not show it so much in its female population, who are not engaged in any special employment.

Defect of Light.—Next to the apparent determination to exclude fresh air from the habitations of man, and from all the places in which people assemble for the purposes of religious worship, business, and pleasure, is the apparent determination to prevent full access of light to the human body. The paramount importance of light to vegetation, so that through it plants acquire not only their verdure but the variegated colors which we admire in their flowers, as well as their requisite firmness of texture and the distinctive flavor of their juices, seems to have received only a passing application, suggestive of its producing analogous effects on animals. The bleaching and sickly character of vegetables, which follow the privation of solar light, and their sleep during the night, showing greatly diminished vital activity, find their parallels in the influence of the same cause on the animal economy. Comparative physiology furnishes additional proof in the same line of argument. When the eggs of a frog are put in water, in a vase with opaque sides and top, so as to exclude the light, they evince no change; whereas, eggs in water of the same quantity and temperature, exposed to the light, undergo a gradual development, and exhibit in due time young tadpoles. The subsequent transformation of these beings is not prevented, but it is retarded by their being kept in darkness Edwards, who made these experiments, thought that in countries in which nudity was allowed by the nature of the climate, exposure of the whole surface of the body to light, or to insolation, as we may term it, was very favorable to good bodily conformation. Humbolt seems to incline to the same opinion. He asserted that deformity and deviations from the natural standard of symmetry are very rare in certain races of men, especially among those with a highly-tinted dermoid system. The sinister effects of want of the sun's light in underground apartments, and in houses, narrow alleys, and in deep courts, almost blocked out from its genial access, ought to share largely with humidity and impure air in the production of scrofula and scurvy, and must count its full share in the etiology of anæmia and chlorosis, and of the pallid and earthy-colored skin of miners, and the tenants of prisons, as also of those persons who lead a sedentary life in ill-lighted habitations. Dr. Brown, of Chatham, near London, calls attention (*Sanitary Review*, April, 1858) to the injurious effects of underground kitchens. He would have large room for comment in some of our cities, especially New York, in which there are not only underground kitchens, but where also it is quite common to meet with dining, and sometimes sleeping-rooms thus situated. This vicious architectural arrangement is too common also in Philadelphia. Dampness is generally associated with the want of light, and performs a not unimportant part in causing disease, by withdrawing from the body, as Dr. Brown supposes, "its normal proportion of electricity, and thus occasions disorders that depend upon diminished nerve force. These are ague, neuralgia, certain forms of rheumatism, epilepsy, chorea, and asthma, with some other affections, such as dyspepsia." The servant girls of London exemplify, in their etiolated condition, and their breathlessness, as well as the anæmia under which they suffer, the evil effects of dampness and of deprivation of the solar rays. The functions peculiar to their sex are carried on imperfectly, or are absolutely suspended; hence the headache, the pains in the side, the palpitation, and the dropsical ankles so frequently witnessed in this class. Organic disease of the heart is originated by these causes in some instances. Another consideration stated by Dr. Brown, but not bearing on our present theme, is the exhaustion attendant on the frequent ascent and descent of stairs.

Dr. Elisha Harris, in his replies to the New York Committee, lays great stress on the privation of sunlight to a vast proportion of the population of the city, "not only in workshops, in warehouses, in counting-rooms, and in basements; but in the modern tenement-houses, the hotels, the school-rooms, the churches, and the private dwellings." He adds, and with becoming warmth of language: "So important is light to human health, that it should be made a legal offense for any party to deprive a neighboring dwelling of light." He repeats an observation of Sir John Wylie, for many years physician to the Emperors Alexander and Nicholas, of Russia, viz.: that in a certain barrack at St. Petersburg, the mortality on the dark side, that from which sunlight was always excluded, was two hundred times greater than on that side on which the sun shone, and penetrated into the windows and doors of the apartments.

THE REMEDIES.—After a tolerably full notice of the impurity, and, still worse, the virulent properties and effects of the air, caused by overcrowding and defective ventilation, we are the better prepared to inquire into the means of the cure, and still better, because acting on a larger scale, the prevention of the evils described. The measures for meeting this object must be undertaken and carried out on a scale commensurate with the extent of the obstructions to be overcome. They require for their successful performance, discreet but firm legislation. First should be carried into effect the recommendation of the English commissioners already noticed, viz.: to empower the local and municipal administrative bodies, to raise money for the purchase of property, with a view of opening thoroughfares and widening streets, courts, and alleys, so as to improve the ventilation of the densely-crowded districts of towns, as well as to increase the general convenience of traffic. Practical suggestions in this line occur to us on learning the steps taken by the present Emperor of France, for the improvement and embellishment of Paris. There may be a difference of opinion respecting the motives which influence the French ruler in the great changes which have been brought about, and others still in progress and projected, in the interior of the capital; but of one thing we may be well assured, that the public health will gain immensely, and this through the external ventilation procured by the new wide and magnificent streets, which intersect, and, in degree, break up the crowded dens of miserable tenements, in dark and narrow streets, occupied by a population ready at any hour to engage in scenes of public revolution or of local outbreak and bloodshed. With a view of securing better ventilation, the Commissioners farther recommended, that courts and alleys be not built of a less width than twenty feet, to be open at both ends; and that they have an opening of not less than ten feet from the ground upwards, at each end; the width of the court being in proportion to the height of the houses. Streets are not to be of less width than thirty feet.

Local acts, as authorized by acts of Parliament, have already been passed in Liverpool, Leeds, and London, and doubtless in other cities and towns, since our attention was last directed to this point, prohibiting the use of cellars in dwellings, unless they are so constructed as to provide protection against the existence of the evils which we have just pointed out. The Commissioners farther recommended that, after a limited period, the use of cellars as dwellings be prohibited, unless the rooms are of certain dimensions, and are provided with a fire-place, and window of sufficient size, made to open, and that said dwelling have an open space in front; and also, that the foundation be properly drained. Prohibitions have been suggested, if not laid down by actual enactment, against building houses back to back—a vicious practice, which effectually prevents both a deep supply of light, and any adequate ventilation by a through current of air through each house.

"The French Government has appropriated 10,000,000 francs to encourage the building of workmen's dwellings. Many model cottages are now being erected in the neighborhood of Paris; each is designed for four families, and each containing four rooms, is to be let at 150 francs a year. They are to be exclusively for laboring men and their families, and to be supplied with water and gas. One hundred and fifty more of these chalets are to be erected in and about Paris; and already 15,000 applications have been made for them to the Administration.

"At Mulhouse, a society had expended, up to the close of 1855, 900,000 francs, for a like object; the Government having contributed 150,000 francs.

"At Genoa, where the municipality expended 12,500,000 francs, during the last invasion of the Cholera, chiefly for the relief of those living in defective, unhealthy dwellings, a company has been formed to erect houses for workmen, in which the King of Sardinia has taken 150 shares.

"At Berlin, there is a Building Society, under the patronage of the Prince of Prussia, with a capital of 200,000 thalers, which yields 4 per cent. on the investment. It has now 202 occupied dwellings, and 27 work-shops.

"In Tuscany, the Grand Duke, in October, 1844, issued a decree, empowering all municipal magistrates within his territory, who may deem it expedient, to form a commission for providing the means of cleansing and rendering wholesome the dwellings actually let or occupied by any other person than the proprietor, which are in such a state as to be dangerous to the health of the occupants or community.

"There are also societies to improve the dwellings of the working men at Parma, Dresden, Brandenburg, Bremen, Chemnitz, Locle in Switzerland, and many other places.

"The houses erected are incomparably better than the ordinary dwellings for the same class; the rents are lower, with the privilege generally to the tenants of becoming proprietors."*

Model Houses.—After State and municipal governments shall have done their duty, by wise and liberal enactments, and providing means for giving them effect, a large field will still be left for the exercise of individual benevolence, or of voluntary associated effort, to carry on a series of auxiliary measures, which are necessary to the completion of those of a public and administrative nature. Among these it is pleasant to be able to announce, not merely the inception of plausible plans but their already successful execution, as in the erection of model-houses in town, and model-cottages in the country, for the use of the working classes in England. The new buildings, though small, are on a footing of comfort and sanitary arrangements, as to a due supply of water, warming, and ventilation, equal, if not superior, to larger mansions inhabited by the wealthy. The trials so far verify a remark made by the Rev. Mr. Girdlestone, who has taken an active and praiseworthy part in sanitary reform: "that one of the most efficacious means of elevating the condition of the laboring classes is the improvement of their dwellings." At Birkenhead, opposite Liverpool, dwellings have been erected in a style so neat as to approach to elegance, by the Dock Company, for the accommodation of the workmen employed in the construction of the docks and warehouses of that new and flourishing town. Tenements have also been erected at the same place by Mr. William Laird, called "Morpeth Buildings," and others by Mr. Robert Hughes; the former consisting of sixty-four, the latter of seventy dwellings. The first is built on the Scotch plan, in flats, or suites of rooms on a floor, and constitute eight blocks, each block consisting of eight dwellings. The blocks

* The Fourteenth Annual Report of the New York Association for Improving the Condition of the Poor, for the year 1857.

are four stories high, with no yard or cellar, and each flat is divided into two dwellings. Each dwelling consists of three rooms—kitchen, parlor, and bed-room, or two bed-rooms. The kitchen is provided with a range and oven. Separated from the kitchen, by a well-fitting door, is a water-closet, with an abundant supply of water for this and all other purposes. Through the centre of each block, from top to bottom, runs a square shaft, containing the water and gas-pipes belonging to the eight dwellings. A small iron door, about ten inches square, is fixed to one corner ot a recess, close to the ground, through which all the dust and dirt are swept; the dust-shaft receives the dust from all the eight dwellings by eight similar openings, and decends to a very large dust cellar beneath the level of the house, from which it is removed at stated periods. Each house is ventilated by two air-bricks—that is, a space equal to the size of a brick is left open for the admission of air, covered within and without by an iron grating, and capable of being closed by an iron shutter, if necessary. One of these openings is placed near the ceiling, for the escape of vitiated or heated air. There is only one appliance, external to the person, wanting in these houses, viz.: the bath. In New York, tenements of this description have been constructed; and, where ground is so valuable, and the population so dense, in some of the worst districts, they must be regarded with favor, although they may allow of but comparatively limited external ventilation.

Model lodging-houses have likewise been built in London and other places with the most satisfactory results. The houseless, the destitute, and the very poor are comfortably lodged; at the same time that they escape the contamination both of disease and vice, for a very small sum, but which is remunerative to the proprietor. At a meeting, some years back, of the "*Society for Improving the Condition of the Working Classes,*" Prince Albert presiding, it was stated by

Lord Ashley, that the new lodging-houses gave nightly lodging, with every accommodation for cleanliness and decency, at the rate of four pence (eight cents) a night; so entire was the success and so remunerative was the profit obtained, that upon a sum of about 13,000 or 14,000 pounds sterling (65,000 to 70,000 dollars) expended on these lodging-houses, they were now receiving an income of very nearly 1500 pounds, or (7500 dollars) a year. Great improvements have been brought about in common lodging-houses throughout the kingdom by Lord Graftenbury's act, as it is called.

With such examples of successful sanitary reform before them, the people of the city of New York need not hesitate day before entering on a similar course, and thus regain high health-rate which it once enjoyed, realizing the benefits due to its naturally favorable situation, and to certain hygienic measures which have been completed on a large scale at great cost. In the words of the Committee of Investigation of the health department of the city of New York, we can say: "A healthful river flows beneath its streets and avenues, supplying every habitation with sufficient water to allay thirst, to prepare food, and to promote cleanliness. The island on which it stands is laved by two noble rivers, whose tides uplift and cleanse the respective streams. Its sewerage is advancing with rapid stretches from street to street, and the fresh breezes from the ocean temper the coldness and moderate the heat of its climate."

Means of Ventilation.—When persons speak of the necessity of fresh air for health, they are not always aware of the various purposes which it serves in the animal economy. It is a "thing," a substance to be weighed and measured as we would water. It is a food, the introduction of which into the lungs is more necessary than that of the substances commonly reckoned as food which are introduced into the stomach. The call for the aerial food is incessant, allows of no pause;

that for the solid and liquid food is periodical and allows of postponement for many hours. Using the terse language of a recent writer, when speaking of the air: "It affords mechanical support; it is a heat-modifying medium; it swallows all gases exposed to it; it supplies a food to man, out of which he is in part built up; it feeds him with the active principle by which the warmth of his body is sustained. The chief sustaining element of the air inspired in breathing, is the oxygen, which forms a fifth part of the whole of the atmospheric sea." The minute terminations of the branches of the bronchiæ, themselves ramifying from the windpipe, and called air-cells, amount to about six hundred millions. The air in these cells, and chiefly its oxygenous portion, permeates their sides and enters those of the minute blood-vessels, which are ramified over them, and thus finds entrance into the blood with which it mixes, and which it so changes as to fit this vital fluid for the nutrition and building up of the new and assisting to remove the old materials of the organs. While the blood is thus changed by the introduction of oxygen, it gives off, at the same time, its gaseous refuse in the form of carbonic acid and animal exhalations. There is no tampering with the respiratory wants: the lungs must have their due supply of pure air, or the entire animal organism suffers—the lungs suffer, the heart suffers, the brain suffers, and the mind works slowly; the stomach is weakened in its functions; muscular movement is enfeebled; the senses are dull; the natural color of health is replaced by pallor. The movements of inspiration and expiration, which make up respiration, constitute the natural ventilation of the living frame. This living ventilation is carried on unceasingly from birth to death, by the infant as well as by the adult, by the profoundest philosopher as well as the solitary artisan in his close polluted atmosphere, or by the sailor nursed amid storms, in a pure and invigorating air. Whether the circumambient air be pure or pestilential, we drink of it twenty times a minute; if of the latter kind, we look old in our youth; if of the former, we maintain the appearance of youth in old age. The average chance of living to the proverbial age of threescore years and ten may be considered the measure of the purity of the air we breathe.*

Different Modes.—All the different modes for ventilation are reducible to three heads: 1. To ventilate by heat, or by a chemical process. 2. By pumping, or a mechanical process. 3. By the pressure and movements of the atmosphere without let or hindrance.† Dr. Reid, both in his work before mentioned and in his Report to the Commissioners on the Northern Coal Mine Districts, enters fully into this interesting question, which he presents under the following aspect: "Ventilation depends essentially on three conditions: the quality of the external air; the quantity that can be made to flow through it in a given time, including the mode of distribution and the regulation of which it is susceptible, whether in regard to the temperature communicated to it, or the force with which it impinges on the system; and its freedom from any noxious ingredients that may be developed by lamps, candles, fire-places, or by any other special cause. Where sanitary measures have secured the purity of the external atmosphere by effective drainage, cleansing, and prevention of nuisances, one-half of the remedy may be secured, and without such measures no system of ventilation can be successful." "Were it generally known," writes Dr. Reid, "that the movement from an ascending current from lamps is always accompanied in non-ventilated apartments by a proportionate descent of vitiated air, which may have previously supported combustion, and that the descent, though limited at first,

* Dr. Hutchinson. Jour. of Pub. Health, vol i.

† Sanitary Review, vol. ii. p. 208.

may suddenly reach the floor, greater anxiety would be manifested to give vent to such products by a superior aperture." Dr. Guy very justly remarks that no system of ventilation can come into general use which does not prevent draughts, which is not cheap, and which interferes to any great extent with existing structural arrangements.

The great number of plans for ventilation would imply that an easy and efficient system is not yet reached. They are, however, encouraging, as they afford evidence of an increasing desire to become acquainted with the subject, and to give it a practical bearing. The extension to which this report has already unexpectedly reached, will forbid my entering into details, or even repeating the outlines of all the different plans which I gave some years back (1850), in a report on Public Hygiene, read before the College of Physicians of Philadelphia.

Beginning with the third head of the plans of ventilation, which looks to the natural movements of the air by a simple interchange between that of the interior of a house or other building, and the external atmosphere, Dr. Reid thinks, that a well-constructed window, capable of being opened above and below, realizes, when the fire-place is well arranged, all the essential conditions for effective ventilation, in the apartments or tenements occupied by the poorer classes. This, as he admits, however, will only answer when the weather is not severe. It also assumes, what in our towns now is becoming a rare thing, viz.: an open fire-place. This last is replaced by a stove, or more generally still, by a register for the admission of warm air from the air-chamber heated by the furnace below.

One of the simplest, and at the same time a most gentle and efficient mode of ventilation, is the admission of external air through a perforated zinc plate, or fine wire gauze, which is to replace a pane of glass in a window of the room to be ventilated. The plate is perforated with 290 holes to the square inch. It, or the gauze wire, is generally introduced in the upper part of the window, and in the place of the corner pane the farthest from the fire-place. Instead of the contrivances just mentioned, the pane of glass might itself be perforated. The fine orifices prevent the air from coming in with a rush, which would occasion discomfort, and they tend to diffuse the air equally and gently through the apartment. No draught is felt unless a person be seated immediately under the window. But the benefit is not limited to the introduction of pure atmospheric air into the room. There is, all the time, an interchange between it and the internal heated and impure air, which thus finds vent and is carried off. The interchange takes place on the same principle with the diffusion of vapors and gases, even though they differ from each other in temperature and specific gravity. It is in this way that Jeffray's respirator acts, by mitigating the coldness of the external air in its admixture with the warm internal air, just escaping from the lungs in respiration. The plan of ventilation now described is recommended by its simplicity and its cheapness. It is applicable to ordinary sleeping and sitting-rooms, in a private house, as well as to shops, in which, owing to the general absence of an open chimney, or any other means of permanent communication with the external air, it is more urgently required. During the first winter in which your reporter had charge of the men's wards of the Commercial Hospital at Cincinnati, he caused gauze wire to be substituted for a pane of glass, in every other window, and the effects were immediate and perceptible, both in a diminution, if not entire exclusion, of the unpleasant odors which pervaded the wards, the ceilings of which were very low, and which were heated by large coal stoves in the centre of each ward. On the following winter, the gauze wire was substituted for the pane of glass in the other windows of the large ward, and with the best effects. At the conclusion of his first tour of duty in the spring, his colleagues in the Ohio Medical College were pleased to compliment him on what they termed his successful practice in the Hospital. As statistical returns were wanting, one could not attach much importance to this favorable opinion; but if the patients could have spoken, they would have expressed themselves in very decided terms of commendation of the plan by which they could breathe with some comfort, especially during the night, and obtain, at the same time, alleviation from the excitement and pains of fever and inflammation.

Another plan of ventilation still, based on the natural movements of the air, without the aid either of mechanical or chemical means, is by an opening in the wall or ceiling which leads to the external air, and which is protected by a shield or disk, say two inches larger than the aperture. The external air, in impinging against the side of this shield, is split up into a thin circular radiating sheet, and at a short distance below, not more than two feet, a person cannot feel cold entering, nor can the hand detect a draught at eight or ten inches distance from the edge of the disk. The sheet of air may be modified according to the distance of the shield from the aperture. A still farther precaution has been used by Dr. Guy, who adopted this practice for admitting air, through a window-pane of glass. It is to have the sides of a close-fitting shield perforated, and thus to have the air broken into jets. The plan of ventilation through openings with shields or disks before them, has been modified by Mr. Leather, of Sheffield. He introduced it for supplying the day and bed-rooms of the Ecclesball Bierlow Union Poor House with fresh air, and, as he said, in his evidence before the English Commissioners for Inquiry, &c., so often referred to in this report, it answers the purpose admirably. An opening is to be made in the outer wall, and a flue carried from it between the floor timbers, to the middle of the ceiling, where the air passes into the room; in order to prevent the current of air from rushing downwards, the aperture in the ceiling is masked by a large circular iron plate. The purpose of this has been already explained. It is fixed on a screw passing through its centre, and by turning the plate round, the aperture may be closed or opened, little or much, and the supply of air regulated at pleasure. Mr. Hosking, in his valuable work on the "*Proper Regulation of Buildings in Towns*," suggests different plans for ventilation. One of the simplest, and which comes under our present head, is by means of "opposite air-flues, or flues opening to the same apartment, in opposite walls, the flue on one side giving vent to the spent air at the highest level the room affords, and that on the other side delivering fresh air at the same high level." This plan will go far to fulfill the indications previously stated by Mr. H., viz.: the expulsion of foul air from apartments by processes which act independently, and which cannot operate offensively, as by cold draughts; and such processes must be moreover inexpensive, to give them any chance of being largely adopted. The plan just offered will be more complete where there is a fire, whose place is arranged, and whose combustion is fed with air, in a manner previously described by Mr. Hosking, so as to insure its own immunity from ignorant interference, while it requires no manipulation that a child may not supply. For the details of his plan, by which the fresh air from without is introduced behind and about the range or stove, and made to do the double duty of feeding the fire and supplying the room for the purposes of respiration, I must refer those curious on the subject to the work itself. The plan is very analogous to the one recommended long before by Franklin. The air-syphon ventilator originating with Dr. Chowne, is recommended by its simplicity and easy use, and its adaptation to the general ventilation of buildings, of ships, and of mines; and if a little care were taken in providing for its application in architectural designs, many useful results, both in regard to artistic display and hygienic comforts, would be realized. The general principle of the air-syphon ventilator rests on the curious fact, that if a tube of the syphon shape be placed in a room with the long end uppermost, a current of air will immediately play through it, in the downward direction of the short, and in the upward direction of the long, leg of the tube. Another and still more simple process of ventilation is that recommended by Dr. Corwan. It consists in simply bisecting all tubes or outlets by which a current of air is desirable. The bisecting consists in the introduction of a second tube within the first, so as to allow space between the two. If smoke is to ascend, it will be drawn up in a steady and rapid stream on one or other side of the septum, and a downward current more or less active will be established in the other. "Smoky chimneys, for example, with their legionary train of evils and inconveniences, would be impossible, were their spaces properly subdivided; for no disproportion in the relative strength of either upward or downward currents would prevent their independent establishment. The short and ever-smoking chimneys of small tenements and upper chambers might thus be made efficient; and in cases where bisecting the tube was impracticable, suspending a central tube would probably succeed. The pipings of stoves, if so constructed, would be far more certain in their action, while the downward draught could be easily converted into an efficient bellows for the fire." Mr. McKennell, of Glasgow, has constructed his patent ventilator on this system. "It consists mainly of air-tubes arranged concentrically, the inner discharging the vitiated air, while the fresh supply flows down the outer tube. It is almost automatic in its action, requiring little or no attention in ordinary circumstances. It removes the air as it is vitiated, and supplies its place with pure air in the exact amount required, in currents so gentle as to be scarcely perceptible."

Mr. Roberton describes the mode of ventilation of the hospital at Bordeaux, which is on the same principle as that advocated by Mr. Hosking. It consists in having isolated wards, and these open to the air, from side to side and from end to end, by means of long windows, so that a current of air is always passing through, in correspondence with the natural laws of the atmosphere. In carrying out this, the natural plan of ventilation, the perforated zinc or glass plates are most useful.

Under the head of mechanical or physical means of ventilation, come wind-sails, chiefly used on board ship, the bellows or pump, the fan and the screw. The fanner and screw may be looked upon as modifications of the same instrument. All these mechanical plans are described by Dr. Hutchinson, in the *Journal of Public Health*, vol. ii. In this connection, reference may be made to Dr. Arnott's single ventilating pump, his gasometer ventilating machine—in fact, an air-pump—also his double-current warming ventilation. In the Niger expedition, the steamers were ventilated after a plan proposed by Dr. Reid, which rested in the plenum and vacuum principles. A fanner or ventilating machine was put in motion either by the machinery of the steam-engine, or by the "kroomen," or when in the rivers, the paddles being disconnected from the engine, by the paddles themselves, which acted as water-wheels. From the ventilator a series of tubes extended to all the compartments of the vessel. When the fanner worked on the "*vacuum principle*," the vitiated air was drawn by it from the various compartments, and was discharged at an opening in the circumference of the fan-box. When the "*plenum principle*" was resorted to, the fresh external air was connected with the centre, and blown into the distribution tubes to the several compartments. By these means it was hoped that, under any circumstances, fresh air might be infused into, or vitiated air extracted from, the hold, or any part of the vessel. At some periods of the voyage, the air was drawn through a medicator, with the intention of removing carbonic acid, and of evolving chlorine.

Chemical Ventilation.—For nearly all useful purposes, and as an agent, in some sort, always present, and readily brought into play, heat is the most efficient agent, and it is that which gives rise to *chemical ventilation.* In fact, the questions of warming and ventilating apartments are closely related and interwoven one with another. There can be no ventilation where there is no movement of air, and this movement, apart from some mechanical contrivances of very limited use and power, is always imparted by heat; one portion of air rarefied by heat, rising and being replaced by a cooler one, and so on. As long as we have a fire we have a ventilator; and when the difference between the temperature of a room or hall of any description, and that of the outer air, is not enough to cause an active movement of the air, or where this is mixed with much watery vapor or gases, it is necessary to procure the aid of artificial heat, or a fire, in order to give the requisite movement to the air, and thus insure ventilation. With this view a fire is made in the upper part of the tower of a building to be ventilated, and flues are constructed to establish a communication between the room or hall in which persons are assembled, and the chimney of the fire-place, or a common central flue contiguous to and heated by this fire. A few large gas-burners will answer the purpose of this last, and with less trouble to the attendants, and less risk to the building. The impure air is by this means drawn, as it were, from the various rooms below, through the prepared apertures at the upper part, or near the ceiling, and passes along the flues which converge at the central flue, whence it finds its way into the open air, at such a height, and with such a rapidity of movement, as to insure its diffusion through the atmosphere, without its exerting any injurious effects on the people out of doors, or, in fact, without the possibility of its reaching them. By methods of this kind, we could ventilate all places in which people congregate for any length of time, as churches, schools, and lecture-rooms, courts of justice, concert, and dancing-rooms, and theatres, or in which a number of persons are confined from infirmity or sickness, as in hospitals and other asylums, or for crimes, as in prisons. The ingress air, or that from without, is to be introduced in quantity bearing a relation to the number of persons assembled, and to the quantity of egress air through the discharging flues. When, however, it is necessary to procure artificial warmth for the comfort of the parties assembled, in any of the ways just mentioned, then the heating apparatus will rarefy the air sufficiently to insure, after it has been used in respiration, its rising and being carried off by exit flues opening into the external atmosphere. These flues for egress air should be somewhat of a valvular form, because air, except under a powerful and quick motion, will, from any cause, regurgitate into the apartment or hall. By the *internal valve for egress air*, we must be understood to mean some valvular machine opening into a heated chimney-flue, which may pass up the side of the chamber. The internal valve is, therefore, chiefly applicable to private rooms or buildings constructed on a similar system. More than sixty years ago, Franklin spoke of the advantageous system of making a communication into a smoke-flue near the ceiling of the wards of the Pennsylvania Hospital, and that such an opening, together with another in each door of the ward, made them all "perfectly sweet."

The ventilating valve of Dr. Arnott has got into extensive use, and when correctly fitted up, works well. It is placed in an opening made for the purpose from the room into the chimney-flue, near the ceiling, by which all the noxious air, caused by the breathing of persons in the room, the combustion of gas or other bodies for lighting, &c., is allowed at once, in obedience to the chimney draught, to pass away; but through which no air or smoke can return. The valve is a metallic flap to close the opening, balanced by a weight on an arm behind the hinge. The weight may be screwed on its arm to such a distance from the axis, or centre of motion, that it shall exactly counterpoise the flap; but if a little farther off, if will just preponderate, and keep the flap, when not acted on by entering air, very softly in the closed position. Although the valve, therefore, be heavy and durable, a breath of air suffices to remove it; which, if from the room, opens it, and if from the chimney closes it, and when no such force interferes, it shuts. The valve is so regulated originally, as to settle always in the closed position. An important part of the arrangement is the wire, which descends like a bell-wire, from a valve to a screw or peg fixed in the wall within the reach of a person's hand, by acting on which the valve may be either entirely closed, or left free to open in any desired degree. In cold weather, or with few persons in the room, the valve, when only opened a little, allows as much air to pass as is requisite. A flap of thirty-six square inches area is large enough where there is a good chimney draught, for a full-sized sitting-room with company. It is essential for the successful working of this ventilating valve, that the chimney draught be uniform and good, so that no more air shall enter at the chimney-flue over the fire, than can escape at the chimney-pot above. Where the room is warmed by a stove or by furnace, there is less probability of any obstacle of this kind to the chimney taking in air at the ventilating valve.

Mr. Ewart has constructed a more simple, and it is alleged, effective valve, than Dr. Arnott, for the small cost of a sum not exceeding a dollar. The valve is composed of oiled silk, on a frame, on which are six large openings, admitting the egress of air with great freedom. Very similar to this contrivance, is one also suggested by Dr. Arnott. It consists of a square iron tube of from three to six inches in diameter, and so long that the outer orifice shall be flush with the wall of the apartment, and the inner one enter the chimney. These tubes are usually from four to six inches in length. At the orifice entering the room, there is either a plate of perforated zinc or a piece of fine wire-work, from the upper and back part of which hangs a piece of ordinary or oiled silk, which acts as a valve, so as to allow the warm and vitiated air to pass up the chimney, and to prevent any smoke from entering the room. The annoyance of a smoky chimney is removed by this mechanism. When it is found necessary to close up the valve, either upon lighting the fire, or in cold weather, or when a room is first inhabited, or finally, if the chimney should be on fire, a slide connected with the tube can be drawn up and cover the whole aperture.

In constructing a house, Dr. Hutchinson recommends the introduction of a sufficient flue for air. All chambers should receive the air below the level of the head of the inhabitant, and this air should be carried away at the highest point of the chamber, in the ceiling or immediately below it. This direction is not applicable to the flues through which heated ingress air from furnaces, or analogous heating apparatus by steam or hot water below, finds its entrance into a room. Its diffusion takes place without difficulty. Supposing, as is the case in summer, that no movement is communicated to the air by internal heat, and no external supply is obtained by heated air which had just come from the external atmosphere, then must the ingress air be low down; and while entering it should be dispersed or broken up into small streams or thin sheets, as previously recommended, so that no draught can be felt by the inmate of the chamber. It is necessary that the air should be admitted imperceptibly, and thus receive the natural radiant heat of the chamber as quickly as possible.

Perforated floors were adopted by Dr. Reid, in the House of Commons; this again being covered by hair cloth, so that the supply of air be broken up into small currents. The objections to this arrangement were found to be, that the air not only brought with it all the dust and dirt and taint from the feet, but it was likewise directed upon this part of the body, thus increasing the discomfort of "cold feet," from which many persons suffer. In large buildings, as churches, where there is generally underground convenience for directing the air through some favorable quarter below the floor, into the body of the building, and that in particular spots, not near the feet, as in the aisle, this system of perforated floors may be found to answer. In private rooms, there remains only the side-wall for ingress air, and the place recommended in preference, is the top of the skirting board which surrounds the room. But even here some of the objections occur which intervene with the plan of perforated floors, viz., the escape of dust which would adhere to the borders of the slit, if not partially obstruct it, and be impelled at other times into the room by the draught of the ingress air. This latter may be broken into a sheet-like form by other means, which have been already mentioned. Corresponding with the passage round the lower part of the room for ingress air, and free from the objections brought against this, is another passage for the egress air made by openings just below the cornice, which communicate with the external air, and are wide enough to answer the desired purpose without interfering with the ornamental character of the cornice, or the general style of the finest apartment.

Among the latest and most valuable for efficiency and general applicability, is the plan of ventilation of dwellings and other edifices, suggested and put in execution by Dr. J. H. Griscom, of New York. It pertains to the "chemical method, the motive power of the air being heat, but requiring no extra expenditure of fuel, the heat used for the purpose being only the waste heat of the furnace by which the house is warmed. The arrangement consists in the construction of independent ventilating flues in the walls of the house, in proximity to the hot-air tubes, so that the two may be connected together by means of a lateral or branch tube, by which a current of hot air may, at any desired moment, be transmitted from the hot-air tube to the ventilating flue. By this means the ventilating flues, which terminate in the open air like an ordinary chimney, will be warmed by the hot air from the furnace, when the ordinary hot-air register is closed, as at night in a dwelling, or in a school-house after school hours.

If properly constructed, of brick, or smooth stone, the walls of a flue will, after a current of hot air has passed through it a short time, become sufficiently heated to rarefy the air within, thus giving the flue a good ventilating power, even after the current of hot air has been withdrawn. For example, if the hot-air register of a parlor be closed at ten o'clock at night, and the heat, instead of being thrown back into the furnace, is allowed to pass through the lateral tube into the ventilating flue, and so continue till six the next morning, it is evident that, during those eight hours, the interior of the ventilating flue must become thoroughly heated, so that the next day, when the current of hot air is restored to the parlor, the heated sides of the ventilating flue will continue to rarefy the air within them for many hours, and perhaps even days, afterwards.

There being no danger of a reaction of the air of the flue through the ventilating register (as is the case when ventilating openings are made in ordinary fire-flues), connections with the apartment to be ventilated may be made at any point, and even carried to the opposite side of the house, between the beams of the ceiling, to ventilate distant apartments. Dr.

Griscom's method has the advantage of being applicable to all edifices warmed by hot-air furnaces of any description, which, in general, are those most needing ventilation. This arrangement may be introduced into many houses already erected, by connecting the hot-air tubes with such of the ordinary chimney-flues as are not used with fire.

One of the principal advantages appertaining to this plan, is the capability of having a *large number* of ventilating flues put in connection with the furnace. In fact, the number may correspond with the number of hot-air registers, and thus any desirable amount and extent of ventilation be obtained.

Ventilation of Schools.—Happily we can now speak of a marked reform in this matter, which began in Boston, and promises to spread to other and remote places. A committee, consisting of Dr. Henry G. Clark, E. G. Loring, Esq., and the Rev. Charles Brooks, under an appointment of the School Committee of Boston, to inquire into the subject of the ventilation of school-houses, and to indicate the means of remedying defects, reported, after the successful performance of their task, that the grammar school-houses were then in a better condition, in respect to their ventilation, than any other public schools in the world. The first-named gentleman of the Committee, who is our colleague on the present occasion, was mainly instrumental by his ingenuity and perseverance, in bringing about these improvements. In Philadelphia and other cities, many of the public schools received the benefit of the visits and reformatory suggestions of the Boston Committee. Statues have been reared, and other honors conferred, for much less services than were rendered by these gentlemen. They ought to have received at least an ovation from the grateful children and teachers in the public schools. Commendatory reference may be made at this time to the very useful volume of Mr. Henry Barnard on School Architecture in the United States. From page 142 to page 165, 2d edition, the reader will find instructive details on the subject of warming and ventilating schools and other public buildings. Among the apparatus for the purpose, Chilson's furnace and ventilating stove, and also Emerson's ejecting and injecting ventilators, are noticed in terms of commendation, such as had been previously bestowed on them by the Committee. Mr. Emerson very properly insists on the admission of warm air into a school-room, as indispensable to its proper ventilation; and he enforces his views on this point, by refusing to allow his ventilators to be put up in any school-house that is not, by some means, supplied with fresh warmed air. He objects, like most people who have attended to the subject, to the use of all such stoves and furnaces as emit their heat through and from *red-hot* iron; and he recommends what large experience sanctions, that when anthracite coal is used, the stove or furnace in which it is burned be lined with brick or stone.

The great and crying neglect of external ventilation in nearly all the schools, both public and private, in cities, tells heavily on the health of their inmates. No adequate, and in most cases, no space at all is allowed for the children to obtain fresh air, and to engage in healthful exercise and sports during the hours of recess from study. Not only are out-door exercises imperatively demanded for the purposes of full respiratory effect by expansion of the chest, but also of allowing the body to receive its erect posture, and the limbs their free play, all of which is prevented when the children are seated, and leaning over a table or desk.

Ventilation of Hospitals.—It has been well remarked by the French authors (MM. Montfalcon and Polinière) of a work already cited—a Treatise on the Health of Great Cities—that the more numerous and diversified are the causes of vitiated air in a hospital, the greater is the necessity for vigilance in obviating its occurrence. Every patient ought, these gentlemen think, to have at least three hundred cubic inches of pure air per hour at his disposal; and every ward of a hospital so well ventilated, that the most delicate sense of smell could not detect any unpleasant odor; and finally, the temperature should be always kept at 60° F. Ameliorating influences, to the extent, in some instances, of entire reform of old abuses, are now at work in the ventilation of hospitals and benevolent and charitable asylums of all kinds. This is more particularly observable in the asylums for the insane, some valuable suggestions and improvements in the interior economy of which have been made of late years by their medical superintendents. At their meeting in Utica, in 1849, they declared it to be their unanimous opinion, "that the experiments recently made in various institutions in this country and elsewhere, prove that the best means of supplying warmth in winter, at present known to them, consist in passing fresh air from the external atmosphere over pipes or plates, containing steam at a low pressure, or water, the temperature of which in the boiler does not exceed 212° F., and placed in large air-chambers in the basement or cellar of the building to be heated." These gentlemen also declared "that a complete system of fixed ventilation was absolutely indispensable in every institution, like hospitals, for the ordinary sick or insane, and where all possible benefits are sought to be derived from these arrangements; and, "that no expense that is required to effect these objects thoroughly, can be deemed either misplaced or injudicious."

The union of mechanical with chemical means of ventilation of hospitals has been recommended. A small power would be sufficient to abstract the air rendered heavy by the carbonic acid, which is accidentally diffused in consequence of being condensed before it arrives at the ventilating tubes. This might be done by means of a ventilator on the bellows plan, similar to that adopted by Hales, or the still more simple one, the exhausting air-pump of John Taylor, for the ventilation of coal mines, which is worked by a regulated power on the principle of clock-work, and with the addition of an apparatus for opening the valves. "The expense of labor to raise a weight every day to keep it in constant action, would be," Tredgold thinks, "much less than the expense of fuel and attention to produce the same effect by fire, the action being more certain. To produce the effect we desire, the best plan seems to be to have open gratings in various parts of the passages, with tubes from each to the place of the ventilator; and the gratings might be provided with slides, so that the action might be confined more to particular parts, as occasion might require." Another important part of the ventilation of hospitals is that of the water-closets. An effectual plan for attaining this end is to connect a flue at one end with the descending pipe of the basin, or with the well below, and at another end with the chimney of a fire that is constantly kept up. Even where the water-closet pipe empties into a cess-pool privy below, this arrangement is, as we know from actual experience during a period of seventeen years, quite successful; even in a case in which, although water is introduced by a pipe and stop-cock into the basin of the water-closet, yet there is no addition of a trap or syphon. It is necessary for the proper effect of this plan, that the lids of the privy below be kept down, otherwise there will be an upward and offensive current of air from the cess-pool, interfering with the draft from this into the chimney, as just described

At this present time two novel systems of warming and ventilation seem to divide scientific opinion and support in Paris. The one is by M. Duvoir, the advantages of which are said to be: 1st. That it insures free ventilation; 2d. That it warms and ventilates at the same time; 3d. That it is cleanly and inexpensive; 4th. That in hospital wards, where the emanations from the sick are offensive and pernicious, such emanations can be borne away, directly from above downwards, by having the upper opening in the ventilating shafts in each ward closed, and the lower one open. The wards are thus constantly swept clean of all hurtful gaseous products. Among other public buildings is the "*Hospital de Lariboisière*," to which the system of M. Duvoir has been applied. Strong testimony is borne by distinguished judges of the value of its action and of its successful application.* The second apparatus for warming and ventilation, is that contrived by Van Hecke. The apparatus for heating the men's wards at the Neckar Hospital, consists of three furnaces in a cellar, which heat air that is distributed by flues to the hospital. The quantity of air heated is considerable, and hence it need not be raised to a high temperature: this, when entering the wards, is not more than 86° to 95° Fah. It acquires the proper humidity by passing over contiguous reservoirs of water. The ventilation is procured by the agency of a small steam-engine placed in the cellar, but its boiler in a suitable place outside the building, which sets in motion a ventilator, that derives its pure air from the garden, and injects it into a strong suction-pipe placed under ground, and running the length of the entire building. This chief pipe is divided into secondary ones, which convey the air to the furnaces, and thence into the wards situated on different stories. The air enters into the wards in large sections, and without producing sensible currents. The impure and vitiated air escapes by flues, which convey it out above the roof. This system may be defined to be, warming the hospital wards by means of three furnaces; mechanical ventilation by propulsion; complete appropriation of the steam vapor, which, after doing its first duty in the engine, is employed to meet the necessary wants of the patients, such as baths and washing. The ven-

* Sanitary Review, vol. i. pp. 423–4.

tilating apparatus propels from sixty to one hundred and twenty cubic inches of pure air hourly for each bed. Registers allow of the diminution of the amount of warm air brought by the different flues.

Factory Ventilation.—Were we to speak of the bodily ills from factory labor, as arising in part from defective ventilation, we should be met by the counter opinions of Drs. Ure, Thackrah, and W. Cooke Taylor, in England, and MM. Villermé, and Benoisten-Chateauneuf, in France. Dr. Ure contends that, from the very nature of the machinery used in cotton mills, it is impossible to crowd the operatives, and especially those, nine-tenths of them children, who tend the open-spurred mules. As respects the growth and development of persons engaged in factory employments, Sir David Barry, in his Factory Commission Report, relates, as the results of personal observation, that many of the girls were beautifully formed, who had been from ten years to maturity in the mills. On the subject of ventilation, M. Villermé states distinctly, after a careful calculation of data, that the great body of those employed in the cotton mills have a better supply of air at their work than at their homes, and better, also, than great numbers of other classes of work-people. Dr. W. Cooke Taylor says: "I would be very well contented to have as large a proportion of room and air in my own study, as a cotton spinner in any of the mills in Lancashire!" We must look then, it would seem, for the causes of the greater proportionate mortality among the manufacturing than among the agricultural population, to the confined lodgings and crowding in the parts of the town in which the former sleep and spend the time not given to work, and to the want of abundant nutriment, and also in a large number, to habits of intemperance. There are, however, some facts recorded which might serve to qualify the favorable opinions of factory life. Thus, for instance, fewer recruits of the proper strength and stature for military service are obtainable now than heretofore from Manchester. Again: a corps levied from the agricultural districts in Wales, or the northern counties of England, will last longer than one recruited from the manufacturing towns, as from Birmingham and Manchester, or near the metropolis.

All classes might turn to useful account, for the purposes of ventilating both the rooms in their own houses and the larger ones in public buildings, the presence of artificial lights, especially those furnished by gas. A truncated cone of zinc, the upper part of which is narrower than that of an ordinary gas-shade, and resting, like the latter, over the burner, will be perforated near its upper border by one end of a tube of zinc, which will at the other end be carried through the outer wall, or else into a chimney, and thus be a conductor for the air of the room rendered impure by the combustion of the gas and the breathing of persons in the room. This mode of ventilation is particularly called for in small rooms or shops in which the air soon becomes contaminated, and exerts a noxious effect on those employed in them. There is one instance of an exit tube for gas, so elegant that it would grace any drawing-room, applicable for the lights over the mantel-piece at each side of the looking-glass, introduced by Prof. Faraday.

Dr. Hutchinson makes an observation which will be consoling to those of us who encroach on the midnight hour while engaged in the labors of the desk. "It is an error," he tells us, "to suppose that gas is more injurious to the constitution than candles; scientifically the common means of lighting, whether by candles, oil, or camphene, are all gas-lights. The work of a gas company is to take from the coal a certain product, and send it to our houses for combustion; when we burn the candle, &c., &c., we do in the sitting-room the work of the gas company, taking from the material the same product which the gas company sends to us in pipes;

therefore, if there is any difference, it is in favor of gas-lights."

Ventilation of Sewers.—This is done, first, by air-shafts, and gratings over them, at certain distances from each other, which permit the escape of the emanations from the sewer below into the atmosphere; 2d, by establishing a communication between the sewers and the rain-water spouts of the houses; but it is necessary to trap these latter, for, otherwise, they might allow of the escape of the foul air into the windows of sleeping-rooms. A common method in Paris is to allow of the escape of the foul air of the sewer through lofty shafts or chimneys, so that it shall be disseminated at a height which would prevent its annoying the people in the streets, and the inhabitants of houses of ordinary elevation. These shafts are placed, as much as possible, in the least frequented parts of the city; but even then the air escaping from them is a source of more or less annoyance. Sometimes fires are made in these chimneys, and thus a strong upward draft is procured, and a large amount of gases extracted. A simpler and more economical plan, is to connect the sewers with the furnaces or chimneys in large manufactories. The only drawback to a measure of this kind is the occasional risk of sewer gases exploding when subjected to flame.

As ventilation is a means of purification of sewers, a remark may be here made opportunely, that water is the best purifier, by its diluting the sewage and accelerating its onward progress; and hence the freer and bolder the flushing, and the more frequently water is introduced into the sewer, the less occasion will there be for ventilation. In Paris the gutters and sewers are flushed daily with water from the hydrants, 2¼ hours in the morning, and the same length of time in the afternoon. With an adequate supply of water, and the impetus derived from the height of the reservoirs of supply, there is no necessity for this system of flushing, if the water which passes through each house as waste be turned into drains, both private and public. Mr. G. Gurney reported, four years ago, to the Office of Works in London, a successful experiment which he had made for removing or destroying the effluvia of sewers. He accomplished this object by means of the steam jet, which produces a current through the sewer and conveyed with it the noxious exhalations which are then decomposed and rendered harmless by their being made to pass through a coke fire as they are drawn off. The objection to the frequent use of the steam jet in the same sewer would be the disintegration of the mortar, and action on the surface of the bricks on the inside of the culvert.

Supply of Water.—One can hardly overrate the importance of a full supply of pure water to meet the requirements of health, whether we look to the individual or to the congregated numbers in cities and populous districts. Water, in an average state of purity, is indispensable for digestion and the elaboration of good blood, as, on the contrary, if it be hard, and contaminated with vegetable or animal matters, it perpetually disorders digestion, and gives rise to the innumerable secondary affections of the kidneys, skin, and nervous system, and an impairment of bodily strength and activity. Next to its importance as a drink is its use for culinary purposes; and, after this, bathing and preserving due personal cleanliness, and thus enabling the skin to perform its important functions, which are so necessary to the feeling and the possession of health. Closely, almost inseparably, connected with its usefulness in this way, is its paramount office in the washing of our garments and household linen. In the house itself it is impossible to remove, without the aid of water, the deposit of dust and fine ashes that arise from smoke, and the air and gases given out in respiration. As a means of preserving public health, which is but a collective term for that of the individuals who constitute the public, water ranks next to air. Unless it be obtained in abundance, there cannot be clean streets, nor can either scavenging, by removal of surface-refuse, or sewerage, by carrying off through underground conduits this refuse and exuviæ of all kinds, be properly performed.

The Report of the Commissioners on the Health of Towns, made about fifteen years ago, revealed a sad deficiency of water supply in nearly all the cities and burghs of England. Only twenty-six out of the fifty towns in which their investigations extended, were supplied with water, under the provisions of any act of Parliament. Even in these the supply was very deficient, and in many of them it only extended to a part of the town; the poorest and most populous portions receiving from it little or no benefit. At Birmingham, only 8,000 out of 40,000 houses are stated to have been separately supplied; and at Newcastle-upon-Tyne, where the Cholera made its first attack in 1831, it was stated that the company supplied about one-twelfth of the dwelling-houses, and that very few of these had either tanks or tubs. In Bristol, containing, with Clifton, upwards of 100,000 inhabitants, not more than 5,000 persons, constituting the most wealthy families, are supplied with water by pipes laid into their houses; the remainder were dependent on public and private wells.

In contrast with these deficiencies, and extravagant prices the poor pay for water in many places, is its abundance in other towns, as Nottingham and Preston, for example. In the former, the supply amounts to 40 gallons *per diem* to each family; and in the latter, to 45 gallons. The intermittent supply of water at certain points in a city is reprehensible, both on the score of time and morals, not to speak of the confusion and quarreling in the crowd of persons collected round the water-stands. It cannot be said of our chief cities, Boston, New York, Philadelphia, &c., as it was by the Commissioners when speaking of the defective supply of water to the poor inhabitants of so many of the English towns: "The present difficulty, and the labor, after a hard day's work, of obtaining water, have a very great effect on their economy, their habits, and their health. The obstacles to the maintenance of domestic or personal cleanliness soon produce habits of personal carelessness, which rapidly lower both the moral and physical condition of the whole population."

The following is an estimate of the average consumption of water, per head, in some of the chief cities, including not only what is drunk, but what is consumed *per diem* in domestic and manufacturing purposes, also for baths, stables, gardens, washing the streets, extinguishing fires, &c. By an inhabitant of Paris, 2½ gallons; of London, 20; of Philadelphia, 30; of New York, 40; of Boston, 43; of Edinburgh, 19; of Glasgow, 27; of Vienna, Constantinople, and Montpelier, in France, 15; in all France, 5 gallons.

Various means, on a large scale, have been adopted to correct the impurities of water destined for the supply of great cities. These consist chiefly in filtration through gravel, sand, and charcoal. Boiling the water, by destroying the animal and vegetable matter which river and rain-water so generally contain, destroys the taste and odor dependent on this cause; but recourse to such a process cannot form a part of public, however useful it may be in private, hygiene. Boiling also precipitates some of the earths which were united with carbonic acid; but the neutral saline contents of the water still remain; and hence it retains the peculiar flavor which was owing to this cause.

The saving, in the less wear and tear of clothes, and in the articles of soap and soda, by the use of soft water in the place of hard, is very great. In London, for example, the cost of soap used *per annum* is estimated at upwards of five millions of dollars.

Water in Leaden Cisterns and Pipes.—A common cause of the deterioration of the purity of water arises from the mode of transmitting it from the reservoirs and main pipes to dwelling-houses in leaden pipes, for the purposes of domestic economy. It sounds paradoxical to say, and yet the assertion is quite true, that the purer the water, as respects its freedom from saline impregnation, the greater is the danger of its acting on the lead, and converting a portion of it into a salt which is there held in solution. When we speak of pure water, we suppose it to contain carbonic acid, by which its solvent power is greatly increased. Hence rain-water readily acquires an impregnation of lead from roofs, gutters, cisterns, or pipes made of this metal. The saline substances, on the other hand, found in spring and river water, impair the corrosive action of water and air, and thus exert a protecting power. Of these, the carbonates and sulphates are the most powerful; the chlorides or muriates the least so. Dr. Taylor believes that if the sulphate of lime forms only the five-thousandth part of water, no carbonate of lead is formed; and this salt dissolved in the above, or in larger proportion, in distilled water, will still confer in it the properties possessed by river water.

Dr. Dana, who doubts the protecting property of the salts of lime, suggests that the changes in the lead is produced by a galvanic action between it and iron, which may be developed by very slight difference in the state of the lead, as where the soldering is with the usual mixture of this latter and the more fusible metals. Dr. Dana proposes, as substitutes for leaden pipes in the conveying of water: "1. Wood wherever it can be used; 2. Cast iron or wrought iron tubes; 3. Copper, protected by pure tin. The use of all other metals, or alloys of these, in the present state of our knowledge and experience in these objects, ought forthwith to be abandoned." Dr. Christison speaks of an "effectual remedy" which has been lately introduced by a patent invention for covering lead pipes, both externally and internally, with a thin coating of tin. Little inconvenience can result from the use of leaden pipes where the water flows through them by hydraulic pressure, as they can be speedily emptied before using the water which comes from the larger iron pipes beyond them. It is only in cases of slow entrance, and retention for some time of water in leaden pipes and cisterns, that the question just discussed becomes a practical one, affecting the public health.

Effects of Bad Water for Drink.—Favored, as the inhabitants of most of our large cities are, in an abundant supply of pure water furnished to them, they are beginning to forget that they ever drank that which was bad, and cannot realize fully the disastrous consequences of the habitual use of such a fluid. Generally, however, people are more easily led to believe, even if they are not themselves fully sensible of the fact, that bad water is injurious to the health than that the air which they often breathe over and over again is a poison. One of the first sanitary measures of a growing and thriving population is to procure for themselves a suitable supply of good water. All the people of antiquity were alive to this fact. The means on a large scale adopted for the purpose both in Rome and Carthage have been referred to in this report. It is not necessary for me to enlarge on this point, and I proceed to mention, as a warning to all young cities, the evils from using bad water, and as an incentive for them to take measures to procure that which is good. When this, our natural beverage, is impure, it proves to be a cause of protracted ailments in ordinary seasons, and in those of epidemic visitations it acts as a directly exciting cause of disease and death. In marshy regions, in which periodical fevers abound, water is deemed by some, on good evidence, to be as actively a contributing cause as the bad air itself. But its malignancy has been particularly conspicuous in the production of Cholera. Dr. Lankester, in describing the three kinds of water drunk by the inhabitants of London, viz.: 1, that of the Thames and New River; 2, that of deep wells, 150 feet for example, below the surface; and 3dly, the surface well-waters, points out the fact that these last contain organic matters "of precisely the same nature as those found in rivers, which are the receptacles of house sewerage and saline matters, common salt, ammonia, the phosphates, nitric acid, &c., all indicative of animal excretion. Carbonic acid is largely present in these surface-waters, and from the pleasant drinking qualities it imparts to them, actually makes the more impure waters the most popular, and the most dangerous." Dr. Liddle, Officer of Health to the White Chapel District, relates the following incidents: "In a street at Salford, containing ninety houses, 25 deaths from Cholera occurred in thirty of these houses, the inhabitants of which drank water from a well into which a sewer had leaked; in the remaining sixty houses, where pure water was drunk, there were 11 cases of diarrhœa only, and no deaths."*

A gigantic experiment, as Mr. Simon calls it, was made involuntarily and in ignorance by the parties who so largely suffered under it, in its progress during two epidemics in the southern districts of London. It is related as follows:

"These districts (comprising nearly a fifth of the population of the Metropolis) have been notorious for the great severity with which Cholera has visited them.... Throughout these districts, during the epidemics of 1853–4, there were distributed two different qualities of water; so that one large population was drinking a tolerably good water, another large population an exceedingly foul water; while in all other respects these two populations (being intermixed in the same districts, and even in the same streets of these districts) were living under precisely similar social and sanitary circumstances. And when, at the end of the epidemic period, the death-rates of these populations were compared, it was found that the Cholera mortality in the houses supplied by the bad water had been three and a half times as great as in the houses supplied by the better water.

* British and Foreign Med.-Chir. Rev., Jan. 1859.

This proof of the fatal influence of foul water was rendered still stronger by reference to what had occurred in the epidemic of 1848–9. For on that occasion the circumstances of the two populations were to some extent reversed. That company which, during the later epidemic, gave the better water, had given, during the earlier epidemic, even a worse water than its rival's; and the population supplied by it had at that time suffered a proportionate cholera mortality. So that the consequence of an improvement made by this water-company in the interval between the two epidemics was, that whereas, in the epidemic of 1848–9 there had died 1925 of their tenants, there died in the epidemic of 1853–4 only 611; while among the tenants of the rival company (whose supply between the two epidemics had been worse instead of better), the deaths which in 1848–9 were 2880, had in 1853–4 increased to 3476. And when these numbers are made proportionate to the populations or tenantries concerned in the two periods respectively, it is found that the cholera death-rates per 10,000 tenants of the companies were about as follows: for those who in 1848–9 drank the worse water, 125; for their neighbors, who in the same epidemic drank a water somewhat less impure, 118; for those who in 1853–4 drank the worst water which had been supplied, 130; for those who in this epidemic drank a comparatively clear water, 37. The quality of water which (as is illustrated in the first three of these numbers) has produced such fatal results in the metropolis, causing two-thirds of the cholera deaths in those parts of London which have most severely suffered from the disease, has been river-water polluted by town drainage—water pumped from the Thames within range of the sewage of London—water which, according to the concurrent testimony of chemical and microscopical observers, was abundantly charged with matters in course of putrefactive change." (Mr. Simon's "Report," p. 14.)

Dr. Sutherland, in his report to the General Board of Health on the cholera epidemic of 1849, says, that the injurious effects of unwholesome water had been manifest in nearly every affected place; and adds, that a number of most severe and fatal outbursts of Cholera were referable to no other cause except the state of the water-supply, and this especially where it had been obtained from wells into which the contents of sewers, privies, or the drainage of grave-yards had escaped. Since that time much additional evidence of a confirmatory character has been collected. Two examples are recorded by Dr. Acland, in his valuable and interesting "Memoir on the Cholera in Oxford"—the parish of St. Clements, which suffered a large mortality in 1832, when the inhabitants had filthy water from a sewer-receiving stream, and an insignificant mortality in 1849 and 1854, when the water was derived from a purer source. The other case is that of the county jail, in which cases have occurred in every epidemic, whilst the city jail, which is not far from the other, has uniformly escaped. The only apparent difference between the two establishments in 1854, seems to have been that the supply of water for the use of the county jail, and of which the soup and gruel were made, was pumped from a filthy well-pool, within ten feet of one of the prison drains. No sooner were the supply-pipes disconnected with this impure source, than Cholera and Diarrhœa ceased. It appears from an elaborate inquiry by the General Board of Health, at the close of the cholera epidemic of 1854, that the contrasted effects of the disease on the people of two large sections of the population, are only explicable by the fact that one division, comprising a population of about 268,171 persons, drank impure water; whilst the other, numbering about 166,906 persons, used a clearer, and comparatively pure water. The two classes resided in the same localities, breathed the same atmosphere, comprehended the same classes, and averaging the same habits of life; in short, placed in circumstances nearly identical, saving the difference in the source whence they obtained their water for drink. The mortality from Cholera among the drinkers of impure water—of water impregnated with the sewage of the metropolis, and containing in solution a large quantity of saline matter, derived from the intermixture of sea-water—being at the rate of 130 to every 10,000; that of the drinkers of the pure water being only at the rate of 37 to every 10,000 persons living.*

In the report on Epidemic Cholera in London, in 1854, by Dr. Sutherland, much interesting information is afforded on the influence of water upon the spread of the disease. The deduction from the microscopical and chemical examination of the water used in the houses and neighborhoods where the disease was most prevalent, by Dr. Hassall, was: "That there is no water supplied to the metropolis that does not contain dead and living organic matter, animal and vegetable. But the Thames Ditton water, supplied by the Lambeth Company, is by much the purest of the waters, while the Southwark and Vauxhall water is one of the worst, and the waters of the other companies might be arrayed in a series between these two." From an inquiry instituted by the Registrar-General, the following results appear: "In 26,107 houses that derived the water from Ditton, 313 deaths from Cholera occurred in ten weeks. In the 40,046 houses that received the impure water from Battersea, 2445 persons, it was ascertained, died from Cholera in the same time. The deaths in the latter districts exceeded by nearly 2000 the deaths that would have occurred if Cholera had only been as fatal as it was in the houses that derived their water from Ditton." Dr. Sutherland makes the following remarks upon these results: "When it is considered that the sanitary condition of the population does not materially differ, except in the quality of the water supplied by the two companies, it is difficult to resist this statistical evidence of the predisposing effect of the Battersea water, and of the loss of life which has arisen from its use.†

* British and Foreign Med.-Chir. Rev., January, 1857.

† Ibid. July, 1855.

The deleterious effects of impure water are not seen in cities or large towns alone; they occur in small villages, sometimes in the solitary farm-house—any place, in fine, in which the pump or draw-well is in the midst of a farm-yard or filthy court; receiving the surface-drainage of heaps of stable manure, pig-sties, &c. How often do we notice, says Dr. W. J. Cox, green, slimy, stagnant pools, in the close vicinity, and affording the sole water-supply, of cottages. Such a state of things does not often occur in this country; but in too many instances there is a neglect to obtain an adequate supply of pure water, the penalty is paid in the frequent occurrence of bowel-complaint, and the sudden inroads of epidemic cholera, which makes its attacks without any other apparent provocation. In the new settlements of the West, the enterprising pioneer and his family often pay a tax in the shape of disease, and not seldom of life itself, from the use of bad water or its imperfect supply; and in new towns other schemes of improvement are tried, before sanitary measures, both for present and future protection, such as paving, drainage, and a supply of good potable water, are thought of.

Dr. Cox tells us, that water tainted with various organic matters, whether gaseous, as carbide or sulphide of hydrogen, or solid, as putrescent vegetable fibre, or vitalized, as algæ, confervæ, hydræ, fungi, infusoria, &c.—is a very frequent cause of severe visitations of bowel complaints during the summer months. Several instances came under his own observation, in 1853 and 1854, of the aggravation of epidemic diarrhœa from this cause. "That water falling on a growing soil, and running off to lie in stagnant pools, is sure to become tainted with animal and vegetable life, is well known; and when to this is supperadded the circumstances of the said soil being highly charged with effete organic products, the water thus collected must necessarily be highly impure, and most unfit for human consumption. Yet very often it forms the only available source of supply." Dr. Cox alludes to epidemic *scarlatina simplex* showing itself in a small agricultural village in the west of England, in August, 1856. There occurred in all thirty-eight cases, chiefly among the peasantry, whereof three proved fatal. Two of these were in one house, the residence of a wealthy farmer. Here the disease changed its character, assuming the worst asthenic type, with intense throat-affection, and, as is so frequently the case, defying all treatment. The persons attacked were a servant girl and three children, the two oldest of the latter of whom died. The younger child and the servant girl recovered with some difficulty. The probable cause of the malignity and fatality of the disease in this family was its bad water-supply. It was derived from a shallow draw-well in the back-yard, imperfectly covered, surrounded by heaps of decomposing manure and cow-sheds, the black drainings from which were constantly flowing over the soil. Dr. Cox examined the water from this well on two occasions, before and after heavy rains. The first analysis showed sixty grains of solid matter (chiefly nitrates) in the gallon, of which five grains were undecomposed organic matter. The second analysis (after the rain) gave the enormous amount of between seven and eight grains of organic matter. The rest of the village derived its chief supply of water from a good public well, situated at a little distance in a large field, and properly covered from the weather.

Water tainted with putrid contents sends into the air a much larger quantity of noxious organic matter than it receives from the air. If we take the Thames river, for an example, where it flows through London, it has been calculated that 4,000,000 of gallons of water rise daily, in the form of vapor, from the surface of the river within the city limits, carrying with it into the atmosphere some portion of the putrid contents of the river.

INTEMPERANCE.—The transition is easy from one noxious drink to another—from bad water (nature perverted) to alcoholic liquors (art perverted)—viewed as the cause of so much intemperance and disease, under a great variety of aspects. As a question of public health it comes necessarily under our notice, and as such alone it can be studied here. We are not called upon to arbitrate between the two doctrinal extremes in regard to the dietetic usage of this class of drinks, but simply to look at things as we find them, and, as in the case of any other form of physical evil afflicting a fellow-creature, either standing by itself, or implicating at the same time the moral and intellectual faculties, to limit, if possible, its diffusion, and to find means for its prevention. The first of these objects aimed at, is done by legislative enactments, enforced by suitable penalties; the second, or preventive, is more certainly brought about by individual will, aided by, and at the same time aiding, voluntary association with others. Everywhere drunkards, or, as they are usually called, the intemperate, which is the more correct term of designation, are among the first victims of epidemic, and also contagious febrile diseases. They are more readily attacked, and more readily sink under disease, than any other class of persons. "The pernicious effects of *intemperance*, in predisposing to the disease [cholera], have been recognized by all writers, in the East Indies as well as the different countries of Europe. What, then, must have been the mischief done by this debasing and life-destroying sin in a country like ours [England], where it has been computed that upwards of twenty millions of sterling are annually spent upon ardent spirits alone?"*

The value of temperate habits among the poor, in prolonging life and diminishing sickness, has been exhibited in the comparison of temperance provident societies with other societies. The Teetotal Society in Preston (of which how-

* Brit. and For. Med.-Chir. Rev., vol. vii. p. 33.

ever, the numbers are rather small for the purpose of any general deduction), presents, as we learn from the sanitary report of the Rev. Mr. Clay, not merely the smallest proportion of sick, but it also suffers the shortest average duration of illness. The annual mortality in the Temperance Provident Society (of London), during seven years, has averaged only 4 in 1,000. In agricultural laborers, in the prime of life, the most highly-favored of the working-classes, it is 8 per 1,000. Among healthy persons, generally, it is rated at 10 per 1,000. Among clerks, at the same age, it is no less than 23 per 1,000.

It will naturally be asked whether sanitary measures, which are admitted to be both necessary and praiseworthy, or preventing the noxious effects of bad air, generated by street and household refuse and impurities, or by a neglect of paving and sewerage, as well as for arresting the sale of tainted meat and spoiled provisions generally, should not also be brought to bear against the abuse, if not the use, of so active a poison as alcohol, especially in its stronger forms of combination. In some countries in Europe the apothecary is forbidden to sell a poison without an express prescription or order from a physician; and in every country he would be looked upon as open to prosecution, if he passed across his counter a poison, with a knowledge that the purchaser intended to make use of it at the peril, if not the cost, of his life. Ought a man or a woman—for the sex is not always ashamed to be seen engaged in such a calling—behind a bar, be allowed privileges not granted to an educated and careful apothecary? But, while we condemn the apothecary for selling a small vial of laudanum, the contents of which, if swallowed, cause insensibility and other alarming symptoms, if not death itself, we can not only tolerate, but give, as voters, and legislators, and judges, our countenance to the bar-tender, whose customer is allowed to drink his bottle of distilled liquor, with a similar risk of being made—dead-drunk—insensible, and sometimes ending his life in this state of insensibility. No terms of censure and condemnation are thought to be too severe on the person who is administering, at stated intervals, a slow but certain poison, with intent to kill; but men generally have little to allege against the person who also administers, across his bar, a certain poison, under the plea of his ignorance of, it may be his indifference to, the consequences. The more violent and acute paroxysmal disturbances, induced by alcoholic drinks, sometimes excite alarm, but the popular mind has not attained to a full knowledge of the subject, as far as relates to its chemical and physiological relations; and until it is enlightened on these points, we must be slow to censure those who still foster, directly or indirectly, the habit of intemperance, by refusing to sanction, or themselves to set the example of, the avoidance of a practice which so soon and so often becomes a habit, and a dangerous habit too.

One important effect of alcoholic drinks, which pervades the entire organism, while it seems at first confined to the function of respiration, is to diminish the amount of carbonic acid eliminated from the lungs and skin. Valentin, Prout, Fyfe, and Vierordt, certify to this fact. Dr. E. Smith speaks of brandy and beer as greatly decreasing the respiration, and the quantity of carbonic acid exhaled. Dr. Bocker found, from his experiments on his own person, that those beverages diminished by at least one-fifth the amount of carbonic acid exhaled. In 1854, Mr. W. J. Cox, from whose paper* we are now borrowing, performed the experiment of collecting the carbonic acid evolved from the lungs of two healthy individuals during one hour, both before and after administering a dose of alcohol, in the shape of whisky. In the first case, the quantity of gas evolved, previously to taking the alcohol, was twelve hun-

* Epidemics and their Every-day Causes, in Sanitary Review, vol. iv. p. 259–60.

dred cubic inches; after it, nine hundred and fifty only. In the case of the other person, the quantities were respectively nine hundred, and six hundred and twenty cubic inches. These facts show, continues Mr. Cox, that the presence of alcohol in the circulating current is always associated with a diminished percentage of carbonic acid in the air expired, and in the exhalation from the cutaneous surface. The blood becomes thereby loaded with effete carbon. An analysis was made by Mr. C. in 1850, of the blood of two *delirium tremens* patients. It was, in both instances, attenuated and deficient in plastic material; containing a great excess, or from six to eight times more than common, of fatty matters. Lecanu found in one case of a sot, the still higher proportion of one hundred and seventeen parts in one thousand. Now, any agent which checks the depuration of blood in the lungs, and retains in them the effete products of the circulation, as is done in the case of the blood of a drunkard, must be eminently deleterious. It yet remains to be determined whether the blood of a moderate habitual drinker is *pro tanto* in a similar state. Were we to draw conclusions from the prompt effects in the experiments by Mr. Cox, we should answer in the affirmative. This writer has, however, no hesitation in urging "the following fact, which has received overwhelming proof, that the *least* habitual excess *beyond* a very moderate indulgence in fermented beverages lowers the vital properties of the blood; destroys the normal tone of the nervous centres; and as a constant *sequela* most powerfully predisposes the frame to the absorption of epidemic virus of whatever kind. Pure aerated blood affords the best safeguard against the attack of any epidemic. But the more perfect system of house ventilation, cleanliness, &c., will fail to secure this, if by the constant imbibition of alcohol in excess, the functions of the lungs and skin are interfered with, their healthy relations destroyed, and their waste products retained within the current."

We have the encouraging reflection in nearly all the efforts and plans of hygienic reform, that as one evil often gives strength to another, so does the abatement of one evil aid in bringing about a similar change in regard to another; and hence, as living in filth, breathing a close and impure air, and want of nutritious food, and of adequate hours of sleep, predispose to intemperance in the use of alcoholic drinks, so will cleanliness, light, fresh air, proper food, and diminished toil, do much to prevent the habit being formed, or to cure it if it has been formed. Judicious sanitary reform is therefore favorable to temperance, as *e converso*, temperance is an indispensable auxiliary to sanitary reform—if only by its inspiring the individuals who are to be its subjects with a desire, and, at the same time, the requisite bodily vigor, to engage in industrial pursuits. Everybody must, by this time, be familiar with the fact of the pecuniary loss to his family by the idleness of the inebriate, and the cost to the public treasury for his ultimate support in the last stage of destitution; to say nothing of the expense of measures of repression and punishment called for by the breaches of peace and crimes committed by the intemperate.

Preventable Diseases and Mortality.—Having exhibited one view of the importance of sanitary measures for cities, viz., that arising from the attention at all times given to them as a necessary condition for growth and prosperity, and the punishment in various ways, and often on a large scale, when the subject has been neglected, we shall next take a more pleasing and encouraging one, and which contrasts strongly with the first. But before noticing some of the beneficial changes in the physical well-being and comfort, and even an improved moral tone, which have resulted from sanitary reform, we have yet to say something on losses of life and money incurred in many places, by the persistence in old abuses, owing more to ignorance of hygienic laws, than to purposed wrong-doing or want of humanity.

Dr. Lyon Playfair, taking the single county of Lancashire, in England, which includes indeed the large cities of Liverpool and Manchester in its bounds, showed some years ago, by tabular statements, that there are every year in Lancashire 14,000 deaths, and 398,000 cases of sickness which might be prevented, and that 11,000 of the deaths consists of adults engaged in productive labor. They farther show, continues Dr. Playfair, that every individual in Lancashire lives 19 years, or only one-half of the proper term of his life, and that every adult loses more than ten years of life, and from premature old age and sickness much more than that period of working ability. Without taking into consideration the diminution of the physical and moral energies of the survivors from sickness and other depressing causes; without estimating the losses from the substitution of young and inexperienced labor for that which is skillful and productive; without including the heavy burdens incident to the large amount of preventable widowhood and orphanage; calculating the loss from the excess of births resulting from the excess of deaths, or the cost of the maintenance of an infantile population, nearly one-half of which is swept off before it attains two years of age, and about 59 per cent. of which never become adult productive laborers; and with data in every case much below the truth, Dr. Playfair estimates the actual pecuniary burdens borne by the community in the support of removable disease and death in Lancashire alone, at the annual sum of five millions of pounds sterling—twenty-five millions of dollars. He would draw attention to the columns respecting the number of preventable cases of death and sickness in Liverpool and Manchester, or in any other of the large towns, to show the immense amount of money which might be saved by proper sanitary arrangements.

Another view of the subject of preventable diseases and deaths is presented in the following guise: Taking the least unfavorable sanitary conditions of a certain number of people living in sixty-four districts, in various parts of England, as a standard, we may call the difference between this and the general mortality as preventable, and make our estimates accordingly. The people now referred to dwell in sixty-four districts, extending over 4,797,315 square miles, and their number at the last census was 973,070, or nearly a million of souls. Although living undoubtedly under many favorable sanitary conditions, yet investigations will lead to the detection of many sources of insalubrity, such as small, close, and crowded bedrooms, and a neglect of cleanliness of person, and in the surroundings. And yet after all, "the annual mortality per 1000 of this million of men, women, and children, year after year, does not exceed 17. Is it not evident, that under more favorable auspices, the death-rate would be still lighter? Under such sanitary conditions as are known, and with all the appliances existing, can we not imagine a community living a healthier life than those isolated people?"* Setting out, however, from this standard, we are safe in affirming that deaths in a people exceeding 17 in 1000 annually, are unnatural deaths. "If the people were shot, drowned, burnt, poisoned by strychnine, their deaths would not be more unnatural than the deaths wrought clandestinely by disease in excess of the quota of natural death; that is, an excess of *seventeen* deaths in 1000 living."

It may be alleged that an excess of deaths over the standard is inevitable in large cities, but, as justly remarked by the *Review*, whose train of argument we are now following, we lack the measure-line between the attainable and the inevitable loss. "In London, during the sixteenth century, the population lived about twenty years on an average, and 50 died out of 1000 living; consequently the excess over 17 was

* **Sanitary Review, vol. iv pp. 87–8.**

33. That this excess was not inevitable is now demonstrated; for, with a great increase in number, the population now lives about 37 years, and the mortality has fallen to 25 in 1000. Is the excess of 8 deaths a year among every 1000 living, inevitable? This cannot be admitted for a moment, if we regard only the imperfect state of the sanitary arrangements which the public authorities of London have within their power. Nor can it be admitted that the excess of 5 deaths—or 22 deaths instead of 17—a year, on every thousand living, is inevitable in England and Wales, with evidence before our eyes of the same violations of nature in every district." Of the 420,019 persons who died in England in 1857, about 328,163 would have died had the mortality not exceeded the standard of 17 deaths in 1000 living. Of the difference, 91,856, or what may be called the unnatural deaths, 18,328 happened in the country, or in the village districts, and 73,528 in the town districts. To extend the argument. Within the shores of the islands of Great Britain and Ireland dwell nearly eight millions of people who "do not live out half their days; *a hundred and forty thousand* of them die every year unnatural deaths; two hundred and eighty thousand are constantly suffering from actual diseases, which do not prevail in healthy places; their strength is impaired in a thousand ways; their affections and intellects are disturbed, deranged, and diminished by the same agencies."

Dr. Hutchinson sums up the loss to the city of London, growing out of the preventable deaths, 10,000 in number, and of the preventable cases of sickness, 20,000 in number, annually, to be, for funerals, medical attendance, loss of wages, and expense of widows and orphans, £500,000, or $2,500,000. In addition to this, he estimates the loss to the community at £1,000,000, or $5,000,000. He charges to the same account the sums that might be saved by the consolidation of existing boards and companies, improved water-supply, suppression of smoke-nuisance, and revenue from sewer-water, amounting to more than another million of pounds, or five millions of dollars. This gives a sum of nearly three millions of pounds, or fifteen millions of dollars, lost by preventable disease and death, and otherwise bad sanitary economy, to the city of London. Mr. Banfield's estimate of loss to the United Kingdom, from these causes, amounts to fifty-five millions of pounds, or two hundred and seventy-five millions of dollars, per annum.

In the single State of Massachusetts an estimate exhibits an annual loss to the commonwealth of $62,000,000 to $93,000,000 by the premature death of persons over 15 years of age.

Of the preventable mortality a large proportion occurs in the early or infantile period. Parents, on the spot, would be startled at the announcement that the probabilities are against their child reaching its second year; and yet in Manchester, Mr. Roberton assures us, in his account of the statistics of mortality in that town, that for every 100 infants born (in the township), upwards of 33 males and 26 females die within the year; whereas in Dorsetshire, the proportions are less than half these numbers. For the next period of life (from one to two years), the percentage of male deaths is 18, and of female deaths upwards of 16; but in Dorsetshire the proportions are less than one fourth of this amount.

In Liverpool, the low sanitary state of which has been already mentioned, the proportion of deaths to the whole population is as low as 1 in 28.75, and the average duration of life is only 20 years. Some have thought that the large emigrant floating population of Liverpool, chiefly Irish, contributed much to the increased mortality and low average of life in that city; but this is a fallacy, exposed by Dr. Playfair, who shows that in both of these particulars they have greatly the advantage of the fixed resident population.

Not only is the mortality much increased by the preventable causes of disease, but the physical vigor of the survivors is diminished by the same causes. The recruiting officers in the county of Lancaster, which used to furnish the best soldiers in the country, complained to Dr. Playfair that the sons are less tall than the fathers, and that the difficulty is constantly increasing of obtaining tall and able-bodied men.

Diseases of the respiratory organs, including phthisis, exist, according to Dr. Playfair, in the great manufacturing districts of Lancaster and Cheshire, to a greater extent than in any other part of the kingdom.

It has been estimated that the mortality among the poorer classes in England might be reduced 20 per cent. by means within administrative control, to say nothing of the abatement or removal of other causes depending on their personal habits, which are intimately associated with those of the first-mentioned class.

In the town of Preston, we learn, from the full and exceedingly interesting report of the Rev. J. Clay, that, while the deaths in the whole town are one in every 29 persons, yet in streets which are described by him, where there is a neglect of sanitary measures, and the inhabitants of which are equally negligent, the proportion is one death in every 19 persons.

The large proportion of infant mortality in Preston, among the working classes—those least favored on the score of sanitary protection—is an evident melancholy fact, bearing on the same argument. With the gentry, the loss is only 17½ per cent. of infant life (children under five years of age), while the operatives' loss is 55.5 per cent. For the whole of England and Wales the percentage of deaths is 39.1.

The average age of deaths, including children, of the different classes in Preston, is still further confirmatory of the position laid down. For "gentlemen," it is 47 years; for "tradesmen," 32 years; and for "laborers," 18 years.

In our own country the subject of infant mortality is one of the highest interest, especially in towns. We would again refer to a valuable paper on this very important subject, by Dr. D. M. Reese.

This gentleman, in his evidence before the New York Senate Committee, asserts, and as we believe on good grounds, that: "Infant mortality in large cities in a great multitude of examples," &c., ending, "and life." (See the Senate Committee, Rep. p. 99.)

On this subject, which is one of such vital importance to the public health in all cities, instructive reference can be made to Mr. Hartley's "Essay on Milk, as an article of Human Sustenance." The writer takes equally strong ground with that assumed by Dr. Reese, and in confirmation of his view, he adduces a certificate, signed by fifty-eight physicians of the city of New York, men of professional eminence and worth, affirming their belief, that the milk of cows, fed chiefly on distillery slops, is "extremely detrimental to the health, especially of young children, as it not only contains no little nutriment for the purposes of food, but appears to possess unhealthy and injurious properties, owing in part, probably, to the confinement of the cows, and the bad air which they consequently have to breathe, as well as the unnatural and pernicious nature of the slop on which they are fed." Dr. Charles A. Lee, in two letters to Mr. Hartley, adduces his personal observations and experience to the same purport.*

Under the operation of improved sanitary measures in the city of New York, the Committee of Investigation believe that the amount of thirteen millions of dollars, the estimated cost of avoidable sickness and death, and the unnecessary loss of five thousand lives per annum, might be prevented, with an effect upon the happiness and morals of the people which can neither be reckoned in figures nor expressed in words.

* Eleventh Annual Report of the New York Association for Improving the Condition of the Poor, for the year 1854.

The following is a statement of the number of the indigent sick who were gratuitously provided for by the public institutions of the city of New York, in the year 1853:

" New York Dispensary	46,338
Eastern "	19,706
Northern "	14,075
Demilt "	9,006
North-Western "	4,964
New York Hospital	3,526
Bellevue Hospital	4,836
Blackwell's Island Hospital	3,034
Ward's Island Hospital	10,794
Marine Hospital	4,938
Total	121,217

" Startling as are the above figures, they doubtless fall far short of the reality. To this list of 121,000 sick, who are chiefly unskilled laborers, of the most destitute class, should be added multitudes of the same class that are relieved by private benevolence, and the numerous organized charities in the city; also those cared for by the different churches and beneficial societies; and last, but not least, the great body of operative artisans, builders, &c., in humble life, whose occupations sometimes, but more frequently their unhealthy dwellings, induce debility, sickness, and incapacity for labor."

" Infant mortality, in large cities, in a great multitude of examples, which no man can number, is caused by the impure and adulterated milk, and other unwholesome articles of food, which are among the necessaries of life. Our profession has ever and anon sought to arouse public attention to this important subject, but in vain. Distilleries in or near large cities would be an intolerable nuisance and curse, apart from the mischiefs of their manufacture of alcoholic drinks, in view of the single fact that, wherever they exist, their slops will furnish the cheapest food for cows, the milk from which is more pernicious and fatal to infant health and life than alcohol itself to adults; poisoning the very fountains of life. So long as distilleries are tolerated in cities, cow-stables will be their appendages, and the milk, fraught with sickness and death, will still perpetuate mortality, especially among the children of the poor. All the artificial adulterations of milk, as by water or chalk, &c., are harmless—nay, laudable, compared with the poisonous supply obtained from cows fed on distillery slops, for to this poison chemistry itself affords no antidote, since it defies all analysis or synthesis—a poison *sui generis*, utterly destructive both of health and life."

The deaths from pulmonary consumption in England and Wales are represented to amount annually to 36,000, of which one half are said to occur in London. Dr. Guy attributes the great mortality from this disease to be owing to "defective ventilation of houses, shops, and places of work. Next to this, in point of importance, is the inhalation of dust, metallic particles, and irritating fumes. One cause, over which the poor themselves can exercise control, is the abuse of spirituous liquors, a frightful source of consumption." The death-rates of consumption are susceptible of being much diminished.

Mention was made, under the head of Ventilation, of the sufferings, from neglect of this matter, incurred by tailors. The economy of a better sanitary system with them is set forth as follows: "If the employers and the men had been aware of the effects of vitiated atmosphere on the constitution and general strength, and of the means of ventilation, the practicable gain of money from the gain of labor by that sanitary measure could not have been less, in one large shop, employing two hundred men, than £100,000 ($500,000). Independently of subscription of the whole trade, it would diminish their working period of life, and have been sufficient, with the enjoyment of greater health and comfort by every workman during the time of work, to have purchased for him an annuity of £1 ($5) per week for his comfortable and respectable self-support during a period of superannuation, commencing soon after fifty years of age."

When speaking of the greatly increased cost of sewers, owing to defective arrangements in their first construction, the amount lost in this way should be put under the head of money that might have been saved by judicious sanitary measures.

In comparing the mortality of the town of Salford, in which thirty-one persons per thousand die annually, and of Manchester, which is still greater, with the neighboring town of Broughton, where only fourteen persons in a thousand die annually, Mr. Chadwick enters into some instructive calculations, which go to show that there are 700 deaths annually from preventable causes alone; hence to remove these causes might insure an annual saving of a sum of money exceeding £40,000, or $200,000. To effect this saving, the main thing required is that the working classes should understand what are the sanitary requirements to secure health and comfort to their homes. The above sum is based on the estimate that there are twenty-five cases (Dr. Playfair says 28) of illness, on an average, to one death. Each death costs, on an average, £60, or $300, including funeral expenses, medical attendance, loss of labor, and the like. The reference to the necessity of awakening the intelligence of the working classes to a correct view of preventive hygiene, reminds us of the advice so forcibly expressed by Dr. Kissam, as to the means of abating the evils of poverty, so as to reduce the mortality among the inhabitants of certain districts in the city of New York. Dr. Kissam says, with much force: "The poor must have good dwellings to live in, and they must have medical missionaries to teach them how to live. They are taught upon almost every other subject than about how to live. They do not know how to cook their food; they do not know that they are poisoned when four or five of them sleep in a room without ventilation."

Sanitary Improvements.—The importance and economy of sanitary measures for cities are evinced in the great benefits derived from sanitary improvements. Hamburg suffered severely from the cholera in 1832. In 1842 occurred a grievous calamity, as it was thought at the time, in a fire which destroyed nearly a third of the city. The rebuilt portion shows that in it due attention has been paid to drainage and other requirements; and the effect was tested in its having enjoyed an exemption from the cholera of 1848, alike remarkable and important. A comparison of the state of the poor, living in the rebuilt parts of the town, with those living in the old parts, showed that not more than one of the former had been attacked with cholera for ten of the latter. Exeter, in England, affords another remarkable illustration of the benefit obtained by the adoption of improved hygienic measures. These consisted in improved drainage, an ample supply of good water in every part, pulling down of old houses, the removal of nuisances, and greater general attention to the sanitary condition of the poor. In 1832, before these reforms were even thought of, the deaths from cholera were 402, and a vast amount of suffering, as well as heavy expenditures, inflicted on the town. In 1849 not more than ninety-nine cases in all occurred in Exeter, and one half of these took place in the single parish of St. Edmund, in a low, unwholesome district, near the accumulations of a main drain from the city, immersed in putrid exhalations. A still more instructive example is afforded by Nottingham. Upwards of 1000 cases of cholera, of which nearly 500 were fatal, occurred there in 1832. At that time Nottingham, like Exeter, was badly supplied with water, besides its being ill-drained, extremely filthy, and very densely populated. The ravages of the pestilence were confined in a great measure, to the worst localities, the higher and better-conditioned district escaping almost entirely. Since then very much has been done for the improvement of the town. It now enjoys an almost unlimited supply of wholesome filtered water. Nuisances were removed, and the condition of the dwellings of the poor improved. The result was, that in the autumn of 1848, although a filthy village within five miles of Nottingham was severely attacked, yet the town remained entirely exempt, nor did a single case occur there until December in the following year, although there had been much diarrhœa during the season—a clear proof that the epidemic influence had been felt—when five fatal cases occurred. In the same line of encouraging results from increased attention to hygienic reforms occurs the example of Tynemouth, eight miles below Newcastle and Gateshead, in the north of England. This town, like the last two mentioned, suffered severely from cholera in 1848–49, losing 463 out of its population of 64,248. Thus warned, active sanitary measures were adopted, and when in 1852 cholera was again epidemic, those exertions were redoubled; and, as a consequence, 1852 saw Newcastle and Gateshead suffering "from the most terrible outbreak of cholera yet experienced in England, whilst Tynemouth, only eight miles lower down the river, was exempt, although numerous cases of diarrhœa plainly showed that over it the choleraic influence extended, but found no congenial soil." Evidence to the same purport was furnished in different cities of the United States during the cholera outbreak of 1849; as, for instance, in Boston and Philadelphia—although the sanitary measures adopted did not imply organic changes, but were mainly confined to the removal or abatement of certain nuisances, domestic and otherwise, cleansing the streets, &c.

As justly remarked by the *British and Foreign Medico-Chirurgical Review*,* to which we are continually indebted

* Vol. vi. pp. 36–37

for so much in all that relates to British sanitary progress: "But far more gratifying, in every point of view, is the clear testimony which the late epidemic afforded of the strikingly beneficial results of substantial structural improvements in averting the fatal effects of choleraic disease. From a large mass of evidence we select the following facts as illustrative of this most important subject: The three model lodging-houses in the metropolis—two of them situated in a most unhealthy district, and where there were numerous fatal cases around—escaped almost entirely. There were a few cases of diarrhœa among the inmates (210 in number,) and only one case of cholera, which occurred in an old man intemperate and ill-fed. The complete immunity of the 'Metropolitan Buildings' in Old Pancras Road, containing upwards of 500 inmates, was equally striking, although within a few hundred yards the epidemic was so severe that three deaths occurred in one house, and the whole neighborhood was severely afflicted with diarrhœa. Of the metropolitan *prisons*, two suffered severely, while the seven others remained nearly exempt. In the model prison at Pentonville, whose sanitary arrangements are good, there was no cholera, and very little diarrhœa among 465 inmates. Giltspur and Newgate prisons enjoyed, the former a complete, and the latter an all but complete exemption, although the district around suffered with extraordinary severity. The case of the House of Correction, in Cold Bath Fields, is, perhaps, the most instructive of all. In 1832, when the number of prisoners was 1148, there occurred 319 cases of diarrhœa, 207 of cholera, and 45 deaths. At that time the drainage of the prison was most faulty, the sewers having in places fallen in and become choked with soil. Subsequently the whole sewerage was rebuilt, and on examination previous to the late epidemic it was found to be in good order. The ventilation, also, of the cells had been improved, and a small open fire was placed in each of the day-rooms. Out of 1100 prisoners there was not a single instance of cholera, and only a few cases of diarrhœa, which speedily yielded to prompt treatment. Bridewell prison afforded equally satisfactory results. In 1832 it was in a most filthy state, and the prisoners were much crowded. Sixteen cases, four fatal, occurred in the epidemic of that year. The sanitary arrangements of the prison have since that period been rectified; and while the pestilence raged on all sides of it, in houses separated only by a narrow wall, no case of cholera took place, though fresh prisoners of the very lowest class were daily brought in. There was only one case of the malignant form of the disease in Horsemonger Lane Jail, which is situated in a district that suffered most severely. The two public metropolitan lunatic asylums of Bethlehem and Hanwell escaped without loss of life, although cholera prevailed extensively and severely within a hundred yards of the former, and the latter was visited with a rather sharp attack of diarrhœa, showing clearly that the morbific influence was there." To these remarkable proofs of the exemption from a fatal epidemic enjoyed by good internal hygienic arrangement, we may add the case of the jail at Taunton, a town with a population of 16,000, during the prevalence of the cholera in 1849. Not a solitary case even of diarrhœa occurred among the prisoners in the jail; which offers a remarkable contrast with the state of things at that period in the work-house, the inmates of which lost by death from cholera 22 per cent. of their number, or 60 out of 276. This last building was low, badly drained, and most imperfectly ventilated; there were numerous nuisances within the walls; the people had insufficient space allowed them, and personal cleanliness was very much neglected. The space allowed for each inmate was not above two thirds of what was requisite for safety. The stress of the attack was in the girls' school-room, in which the greatest degree of over-crowding existed. The prisoners in the jail were much better cared for than the poor inmates of the Union Work-house. Each cell contained from 800 to 900 feet and upwards of air, besides being systematically ventilated and warmed, to maintain an even temperature throughout the twenty-four hours. Moreover, each prisoner had the means of personal cleanliness, and attention to this was strictly enforced throughout the building. The result was that the health of the prisoners remained throughout perfectly good.

A similar exemption from cholera in 1849 was enjoyed by the Eastern Penitentiary of Pennsylvania in Philadelphia.

Pulmonary and Cutaneous Purification.—The consentaneous, and in a measure identical action of the lungs and skin, is not so generally known or attended to as is demanded by the interests of both public and personal hygiene. The lungs and the skin are both of them engaged in the same offices, viz., 1, to evolve gaseous and animal matters, the retention of which would be injurious to the organism; and, 2, to introduce into the blood the vitalizing element, or the oxygen of the atmosphere; and hence both organs, the pulmonary and the cutaneous, require a supply of fresh air. Both of them require also the additional purifying aid of water. The lungs receive their share in the shape of ordinary atmospheric moisture, and how they rejoice in this is seen in the rosy cheeks, implying active pulmonary circulation and respiration, of the inhabitants of the moist climates of England and Holland. The skin receives its share more commonly in the shape of water, directly applied to its surface, as in the process of ordinary ablution, and of bathing; and in some countries, on a large scale by vapor baths. Both the lungs and the skin exact as a condition for the healthy discharge of their functions, that they shall have their air-bath for transpiration, and their water-bath either as simple aqueous fluid or as vapor, to deterge the respiratory and cutaneous surfaces, and to enable them to cast off, in the first case, mucus, and in the second, the perspirable and oily matters. Cleanliness, in its true comprehensive meaning, cannot be carried out so as to meet the wants of the animal economy, unless we attend to these requirements. Our senses revolt at the mere offer of dirty water for drink; but nature displays equal repugnance when dirty, that is, impure air is offered for breathing; and no less injustice is done to the lungs by the inhalation of foul air, in which are floating, at the same time, particles of fine dust, rising from different substances in manufacture, than would be to the skin, if first, ditch or gutter-water, and then sand and dirt, were sprinkled over it. The very idea of swallowing or even tasting the fluid substances ejected as excreta, or thrown off by disease, from the body of another person, or even from our own, is abhorrent to all; and yet how few scruple about receiving into their lungs, by respiration, the impure exhalations from the lungs of everybody in the same room with themselves. But they are doing more at this time; they are inhaling not only the foul air which escapes from the lungs, but also that and the kindred cutaneous emanations of all those present on such an occasion.

Public Squares and Parks.—We make these remarks as introductory to, and with a view of enforcing, not merely the desirableness on the score of pleasurable bodily sensations, but also the necessity on that of health, of out-door exercise in a fresh and pure air, and of regular bathing in pure water, whether it be fresh or saline. Attention to these things is a duty which every individual owes to him or to herself, but unless it be regarded at the same time as part of public hygiene, and carried into effect by proper sanitary measures, the inhabitants of cities cannot meet the requirements of the case, and must suffer if they are not aided by judicious municipal legislation. The opportunities afforded for ventilation are availed of to a certain and too often to a very limited extent in the house; they are more effective in the street; but they can only be said to have received their full, or in a measure their satisfactory development in public gardens, squares, and parks, in which the delicate and the valetudinarian adults more especially, and all those of tender age, may find compensation for their inability to visit the suburban districts, to breathe fresh air, and to been livened by the sight of herbage, flowers, and trees, in their habitual and ever-pleasing livery. These advantages are all easily attained in the spots of the kind just designated, which on this account can never be too highly prized, nor too greatly multiplied. But there is yet another and a large class, namely, the artisans and mechanics, whose engagements are such as to keep them within the narrowest city limits, and who, fatigued and jaded with their prolonged toil, are too often prompted to fly for present excitement and relief to the drinking-shop, or tavern, in place of drawing on the stimulants which nature affords in the cordial of a full measure of oxygen of the pure air of these open and ornamented places. Here they would experience, in addition, the grateful excitement of the senses in admiring the grass-plots, and the rich parterres, with their shrubs and flowers, while seated under the shade of the spreading trees, and refreshed by listening to the falling water of a fountain, while watching at the same time its feathery spray. It is in such places that town rivals the country, and that nature and art join together to promote the public health, and incite to innocent gayety and enjoyment.

Gymnasia and Museums.—But something more is required for the youth, and the industrious mechanics and working men generally, of a city, than space for walking for themselves and their families, important as this confessedly is. Grounds ought to be set apart for gymnastic exercises and various manly sports, under the supervision of competent instructors.

Connected with these grounds there might be instituted museums of natural history, models of machinery, and even specimens of the fine arts; thus creating in the minds of all who would visit these places, associations of the most pleasing and instructive kind. If we suggest these things as measures of health, others might strengthen our suggestion by urging them as an affair of morals.

Until within the last few years, it was thought that there was something in the Anglo-Saxon disposition and character which unfitted the people of Great Britain and the United States for a due appreciation of the benefits and pleasures of public walks and gardens, and of museums and galleries of art; and that if these places were thrown open to the public, they would be injured, if not destroyed, by the Vandal multitude. Trials made on a large scale, as for instance by throwing open the British Museum, in London, and the grounds and the palace, including the collection of paintings, at Hampton Court, to the public of all classes, have dispelled this notion. The following carries with it instruction. On the occasion of a projected chartist meeting at Manchester, which greatly alarmed the municipal magistrates, Sir Charles Shaw, the Chief Commissioner of Police, induced the Mayor to get the Botanical Garden, the Zoological Garden, and the Museum of that town thrown open to the public. The effect was, that not more than 200 or 300 attended the political meeting, which entirely failed; and scarcely a dollar's worth of damage was done to the gardens or to the public institutions by the working people, who were pleased with their share of the entertainment. A farther effect produced, was, that the charges before the police, of drunkenness and riot, were on that day less than the average of that on ordinary days.

Ablution and Bathing.—As relates to *cutaneous purification*, personal cleanliness ought to be regarded in the light of a sanitary measure of the first importânce, and to come within the category of the cleansing of streets and houses. It does not engage attention to the extent that its importance demands, whether we look to health or comfort. The neglect of cleanliness by the colliers of Lancashire, as recorded by Mr. Chadwick in his Report, is, we fear, not without a parallel, either among the same classes elsewhere, or among many others in better circumstances, but whose skin does not tell the tale to the eye so forcibly as if it were blackened by coal-dust. Neither the men nor the girls employed in the coal-mines ever washed their bodies. "Their legs and their bodies, said a witness, are as black as your hat." One laborer remembered that a particular event took place, because it was then he washed his feet. The effects of these habits are seen in the work-house, in almost every pauper admitted. When it is necessary to wash them on their admission, they usually manifest an extreme reluctance to the process. Their common feeling was expressed by one of them, when he declared it "equal to robbing him of a great-coat which he had had for many years."

How many of those who walk our streets, in gay attire too, wear a garment of this kind over their skins? If the external surface of insects be covered with oil, so as to stop up their spiracles, and the skin of animals of a higher grade be covered by a layer of some impermeable substânce, death results. It needs little physiological knowledge to make us aware of the injury done to the functions of a human body, by the skin being coated for years with the secreted, oily, and perspirable matter. The lungs, to which the skin is auxiliary, must be overtasked in consequence, and rendered more liable to disease. That distressing, and too often unmanageable affection, albuminuria, or Bright's disease, is not unfrequently traceable to the imperfect performance of the functions of the skin.

"It might savor of caricature," says Mr. Martin, one of the Commissioners on the Health of Towns, &c., "were it asserted that in regard to the laboring poor, it is only when the infant enters upon breathing existence, and when the man has ceased to breathe, at the minute of birth, and at the hour of death, that he is really washed; yet such a statement would not be so far removed from the truth as it may at first appear. To the great mass of the people, and from dawn to the term of life, the bath, as an article of comfort, luxury, and health, is hardly known, even in name. In the chief cities of the United States a better, and in some of them an abundant supply of water, allows of the inhabitants having bath-rooms in their houses, for the purpose of cold-bathing; and within these few years past, the increase of kitchen ranges and boilers attached, allows of the use of a warm-bath. But the multitude, the masses of our population, both in town and country, are still wanting in these means of promoting health and enjoyment; and we have ample cause for imitating, by our own municipal governments, those in England, which, aided by the benevolence of individuals, have set about the erection of public baths. These, if not actually allowed to be used by all applicants gratuitously, are accessible on the payment of a very small sum.

As yet, the people of Christendom are behind the ancients, particularly the Romans, and even the semi-civilized inhabitants of different countries at the present time, in the general resort to the bath, and the readiness of access to this comfort and solace by the people at large. Your reporter would venture to refer to a work of his (on Baths, &c.), for a variety of details on the subject of bathing, as a part of public hygiene. Warm as well as cold water should be introduced into all bath-houses, both for the purpose of more complete ablution and detersion of the skin of all adhering impurities, and on account of the differences in individual sensibility and vigor of frame, either constant or connected with temporary indisposition and weakness, short of actual disease. Warm baths might be supplied to the working-classes, Mr. Hawkesby thinks, at the low rate of about six cents each, if taken by 200 or 300 daily. By Sir Henry Dunkerfield's Act, the Parliamentary standard charge, for a warm-bath, is fixed at two pence (four cents), and when the bathers are in reasonable numbers, this sum is represented to be quite sufficient to give a profit beyond expenses. Dr. Reid, in his report to the Commissioners, in which he describes the means of ventilating different kinds of buildings, mentions the advantage of a limited supply of water being procured, " during the progress of the steam-bath, rendering cleansing, and the use of the flesh-brush, much more convenient than in the ordinary water or vapor-baths."

It has been calculated that the waste-water of a steam-engine of 500 horse-power would, at an average temperature of 70 to 75 deg. F., suffice to bathe 26,000 persons. A new source of an abundant supply of water, of a somewhat elevated temperature, adapted to personal and domestic wants, has been opened of late years in Artesian wells. The most remarkable of these is the one at Grenelle, near Paris, which, from a depth of nearly 2000 feet, sends up a volume of water equal to 132,000 gallons every twenty-four hours, at a temperature of 82 deg. F. Its softness and temperature adapt it admirably to the purposes of a bath and of washing clothes, for both of which it is largely used.

Public Wash-houses.—One of the marked improvements in public hygiene of late years, and which bears evidence that the spirit of philanthropy is abroad and active, is the establishment of Public Wash-houses, to which women of the poorer classes can go, and have the use of rooms, and all the appliances for washing and drying their clothes and those of their families, on the payment of a very small sum. The trials so far, made in England and different cities of this country, have been quite successful, and promotive of much good and comfort to the parties for whom these houses are opened. Incidental but very decided benefit to the women who make use of the conveniences thus offered, is enjoyed in the avoidance of the dirt and litter, and confusion and disturbance to the whole family, on a washing day, in their own small and confined rooms.

An improvement, or rather an exceedingly useful addition, has been made to the original plan, by the procuring of large, airy rooms in which the infant children of the wash-women who come to wash their clothes, stay, and are watched and nursed by a person employed for the purpose. And yet a step farther has been taken in the way of present as well as future good to these juveniles. It is teaching them the simple elements of learning and morality.

NUISANCES.—A few words may be said on the present occasion in regard to nuisances, a term which in the minds of many has an entirely too limited meaning for the cause of public health, while, on the other hand, some of the more sensitive and exacting would extend the list to an almost indefinite extent. Under the general head of Nuisances are included special obstructions to the public health, such as accumulations of dung and offal, pig-sties, open privies, obstructed drains, pools of stagnant water, noxious smoke and other matters coming from manufactories, and especially the animal refuse invariably found in the vicinity of slaughter-houses, all of which act with so much power in the midst of a dense population. By an Act of Parliament, passed some years ago, aggrieved parties can, by an easy course, procure a removal of evils, when duly specified. The Nuisance Removal and Disease Prevention Act, passed in 1848, with the Amended Statute enacted the following year, are great steps in the way of sanitary reform. They constitute, together with the *Public*

Health Act and the *Interment Act*, a good beginning in a course of wise sanitary legislation, which has already done much toward an amelioration of the great and many abuses by which the public health in England had suffered so much.

French sanitary legislation is more precise, and at the same time, comprehensive, on the subject of nuisances. It distributes into three classes all establishments which are adverse to the comfort, health, and safety of the inhabitants; and it describes in what manner each is unhealthy and annoying.

Establishments of the first class cannot be allowed in the vicinity of private dwellings, and their erection is only permitted by a decree of the sovereign council. To this category belong the manufacture of sulphuric, hydrochloric, and nitric acids, as well as that of various chemical products, melting establishments of fat on open fires, work-shops for the preparation of taffety, leather, and varnished tissues, also of knackers, tripe-men, and cat-gut manufacturers, and of those in which are prepared animal black, glue, Prussian blue, blood-manure, *aiselle* (a kind of dye), and starch, factories of fire-works, lucifer matches, and fulminating compounds. The reasons for placing these together, as the most dangerous class, are vitiation of the air by the disengagement of emanations inimical to health, the risk of fire, and the intolerable odors which they emit. Hence, if allowed at all, it is only within a radius of three thousand feet, after long and multiplied formalities, which want of time prevents us from introducing in this place.

The second class of establishments of the manufacturing kind include those the removal of which from an inhabited district is not absolutely necessary, but which it is fit should only be permitted after a suitable inquiry to show that they are not nuisances. To this category belong lime or plaster kilns, when they are in constant operation, high-pressure steam-engines, gas-works, currieries, tanneries, hat factories, foundries, manufactories of sulphate of iron and zinc, of sulphate of soda in close vessels, phosphorus, imitation jewelry, bituminous matter, chandleries of tallow and of stearine, and workshops for the scraping and cleaning of copper vessels.

None of these can be called actually unhealthy to those in their vicinity, but many of them are disagreeable, and seriously annoy others by their smoke, their noise, the danger of fire, or by their offensive smell.

The third class comprises all those establishments which may be in operation in the vicinity of dwelling-houses without inconvenience, but which must nevertheless be submitted to the inspection of the Prefect of the Department, for his authorization. They are, lime and plaster kilns, used not more than a month in the year, brick-yards, potteries, and tile works, manufactories of gelatine and isinglass, crucible foundries, dye-works, &c.

There is nothing absolute in this classification, inasmuch as that a particular manufactory, the processes of which are improved, may pass from one category to another.

Considering the excessive annoyances from the smoke, especially from the burning of bituminous coal, in large cities, such as London, and some of our own on this side of the Atlantic, it becomes a measure of the first importance, as a question of public health, connected with its effects on the lungs, by its being constantly breathed, and on the skin, in relation to personal cleanliness, and to the interiors of houses, on the score of domestic cleanliness, to discover the means by which the evil can be materially abated, if not entirely neutralized. Experiments with more or less success have been made with this view, the precise results of which, or their relative value, need not be introduced here. Too much importance has been attached to the mere effect of lofty chimneys in removing to a distance and diluting the heavy smoke and noxious fumes which are evolved from many manufactories. In themselves they in no way destroy the emanations which are conveyed into them; these are discharged as much as before into the external atmosphere; and experience has proved that even very lofty chimneys, on which large sums have been expended, do not necessarily insure that amount of admixture with the common air which is essential to prevent the most injurious consequences of their deposit, even at very considerable distances. The extent to which nauseous, acrid, and other noxious fumes from manufactories often destroy the atmosphere of numerous dwellings, and sometimes of whole streets, is abundantly explained in the reports of the Commissioners.

Slaughter-Houses.—These nuisances, of the worst class, were clung to in England and elsewhere, with a tenacity such as might imply a thorough conviction of the use of them being a time-honored privilege, interwoven with the dearest rights of the people. The last and decisive battle of old prejudices against the clearest evidences of hygiene, was fought in the matter of the Smithfield Market and its shambles, in the very heart of London. We cannot introduce the subject better than by giving the following portion of Abstract of Evidence before the Select Committee of the House of Commons on Smithfield Market, May, 1847.

Dr. Jordan Roche Lynch had lived and practised for the last fifteen years in the neighborhood of Smithfield, the sanitary state of which was most defective. The slaughter-houses have a most injurious influence upon the district; they generate fever, and render the most simple diseases malignant, and shorten the duration of life. In Bear alley, a lane running from Farringdon street to the old wall of London, called Breakneck Steps, there is a slaughter-house behind six or seven houses, which are inhabited by the humblest classes of society. The stench is intolerable, arising from the slaughtering of the cattle, and the removal of the fecal matters, the guts, the blood, and the skins of the animals.

When they clean the guts, the matter is turned out; some of the heavier parts of the manure are preserved to be carted away, but a great deal of it is carried into the sewers, which have gully-holes; and in the summer months, the heat acting upon the fecal matter causes its decomposition; and carburetted and sulphuretted hydrogen gas, and carbonic acid gas, all of which are fatal to animal life, are disengaged, and rush out of the gully-holes, so that a blind man's nose will enable him to avoid approaching these outlets. Whenever he goes into places or houses contiguous to the slaughter-houses, he is compelled to hold his nose all the time he is there, the stench is so great. Dr. Lynch has patients in all these houses. They are never free from the effects of this stench, and when the people there are dangerously ill, he is without the hope, by any exercise of skill, of restoring them to health. He invariably makes it a rule to entreat them to conquer their repugnance to go into the Work-house, in order that they may have better air; and if they accede, the medicines that would have failed in the noxious atmosphere before, restore them, in most instances, to health.

The people where such smells are, drink; it is a kind of instinct; they fly to it; they fancy that the stimulus resists the noxious agency of the foul air they are breathing. Malaria, such as is generated in these slaughter-houses, is a narcotic poison; it oppresses both body and mind; and under the influence of this physical and mental depression, they instinctively resort to the gin-shop, which aggravates their distresses, by extracting from them the means of living perhaps better than they do, and it might have been added, also, by the addition, in this way, of one poison to another.*

Mr. Dunhill, civil engineer, who made the abstract from which we have been borrowing, relates also, that in Newgate and Leadenhall markets, the slaughtering was carried on in

* Journal of Public Health, vol. i., p. 244.

cellars, where there was a total absence of natural light, ventilation, or drainage; the blood and dung being sometimes allowed to accumulate therein for months together, or until the pestiferous effluvia caused sufficient alarm and sensation in the neighborhood to originate an indictment. The water supply was utterly inadequate, and was obtained from the most impure sources, while the machinery was of the most primitive and imperfect character. In Aldgate (better known as Whitechapel) Market, the open kennels and water-tables of the wood-way are to be seen almost daily streaming to overflow with blood and ordure. Immense quantities of skins, offal, and dung, were also exposed on the public highway, where thousands of pedestrians were continually passing to and fro.

We have spoken of these nuisances in the past tense, under a belief that they have been abated, if not entirely removed. Smithfield Market has been finally closed.

Some of the witnesses before the Commons Committee, spoke in high terms, from personal observation, of the French abattoirs, which form a striking contrast to the English slaughter-houses. Mr. Dunhill, on this point, remarks: "In Paris, the influence of cleanliness, supervision, and facilities for performance of the duties of the slaughtermen, was very interesting to observe. Their demeanor was characterized by none of that brutality, apparent relish for cruelty, and indifference to the dirt, filth, and disgusting scenes, which those of our own country witness and participate in every day of their lives. Not the least important feature in the establishment of outlying abattoirs is, that bone-boiling and crushing, skin-dressing, glue, gut, horn, and manure-manufacturing, with numerous other noxious crafts in connection with the offal and refuse of slaughter-houses, highly prejudicial to the public health, and intolerable nuisances in the crowded districts, where they are now carried on, would very soon find their location outside the town, in the neighborhood of the depots of the *materiel* which they require."

When the public abattoirs in Paris were completed, they were handed over to the use of the butchers, and all private slaughter-houses were suppressed. Two indispensable conditions have been laid down for making use of an abattoir—first, a copious supply of good water; and secondly, complete arrangements for its being carried away after having been used in the various processes of slaughtering the animals, and in the washing and manipulations of their several parts. Where the water cannot be brought by hand, it must be pumped up by steam-engines. It has been computed that a single abattoir in Paris requires about 45,000 gallons of water daily. The sewers for the carrying off the waste and impure water, are either special, and open directly into the Seine, or communicate with public sewers, which have a uniform fall towards the river. Trials were made, but unsuccessfully, of large pits filled with calcareous stones, for the reception of the waters coming from an abattoir, and also of open drains to convey the waters to the Seine. Finally, an absorbing Artesian well, 570 feet deep, was bored, and in this opening all the bloody and saline water of the abattoir was allowed to flow. The absorption went on at a uniform rate, and without the escape of a single drop of the inflowing water, or of any odor, either inside or external to the establishment.

In the public abattoirs, a supervision can be, and is exercised over the health of the cattle that are brought to be slaughtered. None are allowed to be killed in them which are laboring under contagious disease; nor can the animals affected with other diseases be slaughtered without the consent of the inspectors of the abattoir.

Cow-Houses.—These have become of late years regular establishments in nearly all large cities. Though not directly nor necessarily coming under the head of nuisances, yet incidentally and too frequently they are made such. The subject is doubly important—first, as it relates to the contamination of the surrounding air, by a failure to remove the excremental matters from the stables, and to keep them clean; and secondly, by the bad milk obtained from cows pent up in stables in which ventilation is not attended to. Of the deleterious food given to these animals when kept in stables in a city, and of the consequent bad health and diseases. especially among the infantile portion of the inhabitants of a city, we have already spoken.

Cow-keeping did not elude the vigilance of the French government. The regulations which exist have for their object, to prevent overcrowding of the animals, to insure cleanliness, and a sufficient ventilation of the stables. It appears, from a report of the Metropolitan Medical Officers of Health on London cow-houses, that there are in that metropolis 846 of these establishments, containing 11,818 cows. The Committee, in conclusion, offer the following rules for the regulation of cow-houses:

1. Every cow-house shall be paved with flag-paving or other non-absorbent material, set and bedded in cement, with a proper inclination to the foot of the stalls, so as to drain into a channel leading, by a fall of not less than one and a half inches, or ten feet in a trapped gully.

2. Every cow-house will be provided with a proper trapped drain, to convey fluid matter alone into the sewers.

3. Every cow-house shall be furnished with an adequate supply of water, and be washed thoroughly at least once a day.

4. All solid manure and refuse shall be carefully swept up twice a day, be kept under cover, and be carted away every morning by seven o'clock from Lady-day to Michaelmas, and by eight o'clock from Michaelmas to Lady-day.

5. Every cow-house shall be kept in proper condition, and the walls be lime-washed at least four times a year, within fourteen days after the quarter.

6. Every cow-house shall have at least 8 feet by 4 feet for each cow (when the cows are kept in separate stalls), or of 8 feet by 7 feet for every two cows (where the stalls are constructed to hold pairs), with a cubic capacity, in either case, of at least 1000 feet to each cow; shall be properly lighted and ventilated, and when the state of the neighborhood requires it, shall be provided with tight roofs and ventilating shafts, so as to convey the noxious exhalations above the level of the adjacent houses.

7. Every yard in which a cow-house is situated, shall be well paved with stone, or other impervious material (the joints of the paving to be run with grout), with such a slope towards the channels and trapped gully, as to permit the rapid escape of all fluids into the sewer, and shall be washed at least once a day.

8. The grain-bins and receptacles for wash, shall be kept properly cleaned, and under cover.

9. No underground cellar, and no part of a dwelling-house, shall be used as cow-sheds.

Among the most grievous nuisances to which many neighborhoods have been subjected in London and other large towns, is burial-grounds not adequate for complete sepulture. Indeed, the practice of intra-mural interment, that is, of burial of the dead in a densely populated part of a city, must altogether be regarded in the light of a nuisance. It is not necessary to enlarge on this subject, as it has been made one of separate investigation by your reporter, and as such it is now offered to the Convention as the completion of his labors at this time.

INTERMENTS IN CITIES.

There yet remains one important branch of sanitary reform, bearing on the public health, to which attention must now be directed. It is interment of the dead in city limits. Turning to present account the materials which, as chairman of a committee appointed for the purpose by the Philadelphia County Medical Society, your reporter collected and presented to that body, he now offers this document, with some additions, as a contribution, on the part of the Committee on the Internal Hygiene of Cities, to the Quarantine and Sanitary Convention.

The practice of intra-mural interments, or of those within the limits of a city or town, and especially in those parts of it in which people are congregated in numbers for fixed habitation, is always dangerous to the public health. It has caused, in numerous instances, sudden death; and to a still greater extent, it has been productive either of fatal disease, or of a slow decay of the powers of life, and a breaking down of the constitution. Enlightened legislation, from the earliest times, has endevored to prevent, or if this could not be done, to mitigate the evils attendant on interments in cities and towns. Sometimes a religious sanction was given as the means best adapted to attain these objects. This was the case in ancient Egypt, in which, owing to the nature of the soil and the annual overflow of the valley of the Nile, inhumation could not be performed in a proper manner; and hence the universal resort to embalming the dead, which came to be regarded both as a religious and a hygienic measure. The bodies thus prepared were afterwards deposited in grottos and in chambers excavated from the rocks, the walls of which were covered with bas-reliefs and fresco paintings, descriptive of the trades and other occupations of the deceased. The Etruscans, to whom Rome was indebted for her ritual, her first sanitary regulations, and the construction of the great cloaque, took wise precautions against the dead being a cause of disease and of terror to the living, by arrangements for sepulture on such a scale, that in their excavated cities of the dead, the traveler, at the present time, sees sepulchral chambers so ample and decorated, as to persuade him that he is actually in the houses of the former inhabitants

In the primitive ages of Greece, the inhabitants buried their dead in depositaries prepared for the purpose in their own houses; and vaults in temples were sometimes used in this way. But with the progress of refinement and better knowledge, the custom afterwards prevailed of carrying the dead without the cities, and interring them chiefly by the highways. Lycurgus, in this, as in most of his institutions, differed from the rest of the Greek lawgivers, for he allowed the Lacedemonians not only to bury their dead in the city, but also around their temples. His object was to remove from the minds of the youth the fear of a dead body, as well as to destroy the superstitious dread, that treading on a grave or touching a dead body would defile. Burning the bodies of the dead became general among the Greeks, from whom the Romans afterwards borrowed the custom.

The ancient Jewish cemeteries were commonly situated beyond the limits of cities and villages. It was, indeed, the custom among other nations of the East as well as among the Hebrews, to bury out of the city, except in the case of kings and very distinguished men. The Hebrews generally exhibited a preference for burying in gardens, and beneath shady trees. Large subterranean places of interment were frequently to be found in Palestine: in some instances they were the work of nature; in some they were merely artificial excavations of the earth, and in others were cut out from rocks. Numerous sepulchres of this kind are still found in Syria and also in Egypt. Examples of these subterranean quarries, used probably for the same purpose, are seen at

Marsala (the ancient Lilybæum) in Sicily, Syracuse, Salerno, Malta, and, in the north at Maestricht, &c.; and perhaps, adds Mr. Burton,* the celebrated labyrinth in the island of Crete was formed originally by excavations of the kind. But by far the most remarkable are those discovered of late years by Laborde, in the remains of the large and wealthy city of Petra, the ancient Edom. They are of incredible number and extent, and of various forms and dimensions. Some of them are houses and palaces; but the greater number are tombs and the like sepulchral monuments. They not only occupy the foot of the entire mountain by which the valley is encompassed, but the ravines and recesses which branch out from the inclosed area. Ranged in regular order, like houses of a well-built city, they would extend, we are told by the Rev. Dr. Olin, who visited the place, not less than five or six miles in length. The façades of many of these rock tombs are decorated with great architectural and sculptural beauty; the more striking on account of the utter solitude and desolation in which they are found.

The Carthaginians buried their dead at some distance from the city. The Necropolis was situated beyond the suburbs, or the new town, Megara, as it was called, which, itself, was made up chiefly of gardens intersected by canals for the purpose of irrigation.

In the brightest or the republican period of the history of Rome, down to the time of Sylla, the ordinary method of inhumation was practised in either public or private places. The private were in fields and gardens, often on the sides of the most frequented roads, so as to attract the notice of those that passed, and it may have been also to remind them of their mortality. Hence the frequent inscriptions on the tombs: Stop, Traveler; Behold, Traveler, &c. (SESTE VIATOR; ARPICE VIATOR), seen on the Appian, the Aurelian,

* Description of the Antiquities and other Curiosities of Rome

the Flaminian, and other roads. Public places, such as the Campus Esquilinus outside the Esquiline gate, were granted by the Senate for poor people. The vast accumulation of the dead at this spot rendered the neighborhood so unhealthy, that Augustus, with the consent of the Senate, gave part of it to his favorite Mæcenas, who built on it a magnificent house, and surrounded it by extensive gardens. The Roman law was very decided in its prohibition of the burial of the dead within the city; and only in a few exceptional cases was any relaxation permitted. The vestal virgins and some illustrious men were favored in this way. The right of sepulture for himself within the poemarium, or open space left both within and outside of the walls, was decreed to Julius Cæsar, as an unusual privilege. By the emperors the original law was enforced with a severity which was rendered the more necessary by its frequent infractions on the part of the people, who believed the worship of their household gods and the manes of their ancestors to be more acceptable in the vicinity of the dead. Adrian decreed the confiscation of the land on which a tomb was reared within the city limits, and the exhumation of the body which had been buried.

Burning the bodies of the dead, of which mention is made in the laws of Numa and of the Twelve Tables, did not become general until towards the end of the republic. Under the emperors the custom was almost universal, but it afterwards gradually declined on the introduction of Christianity, and fell into disuse about the end of the fourth century. The Romans prohibited both the burning and the burial of the dead in the city; in the former case in order that houses might not be endangered by the frequency of funeral fires, and the air contaminated by the stench arising from them. The Senate House, contiguous to the Forum, was burned by the flames extending from the funeral pile of Clodius.

The canons of the Christian Church, in imitation of the

civil law, were opposed to interments in cities, and also in their churches, but with indifferent success. The pernicious examples set by the Emperor Constantine, who, in pursuance of his expressed wish, was buried in the vestibule of the Basilica of the Holy Apostles at Constantinople, and by Honorius, who found a sepulchre in the portico of the Church of St. Peter's, at Rome, soon had numerous imitators among the patricians and great officers of the state. Vainly did succeeding emperors forbid intra-mural interments, and endeavor to restrict the privilege to martyrs alone. Mistaken piety, superstition, and the vanity of the rich and the powerful, prevailed over imperial edicts, and before the sixth century there were not only numerous interments in towns, but the practice of sepulture in churches was also on the increase. The monks obtained permission to be buried in the cloisters of their convents, and the founders of churches procured for themselves the same privilege. Charlemagne, toward the close of the eighth century, seconding the wise reform of these abuses begun by Theodolphus, bishop of Orleans, prohibited the burial of the laity in churches, and eventually of all persons whatever. But the evil was not arrested, although attempts were made with this view by numerous great councils of the Catholic Church, held in different parts of Europe, from the beginning of the ninth to the latter part of the sixteenth century. Why prohibitions, enjoined under such solemnity, were so long and so extensively disregarded, may be understood for the reasons already assigned. To these should be added another and constantly nullifying cause, viz.: the cupidity of the clergy, who derived large fees for the permission which they granted to bury in churches or contiguous porticos; and this often in despite of positive enactments by some of the councils against such abuses. Even somewhat less than a century ago, or in 1765, the Parliament of Paris, disregarding the remonstrances of the physicians, who had called the attention of the government to the danger of intra-mural burials, continued the permission to the clergy to be interred in the churches. It was not long, however, before the clerical body, animated by a more enlightened spirit, gave up privileges which were productive of so much danger to the public health; and at the present time the traveler has an opportunity of admiring the numerous and tastefully-arranged suburban and rural cemeteries in France, Italy, and Germany, which have replaced the crowded and often closely body-packed and noisome grave-yards and church-vaults in the central parts of the cities.

The practice by the first Christians of interring their dead in the city of Rome, grew out of the peculiar circumstances in which they were placed as a persecuted sect. As such they were compelled to hold their religious meetings and to celebrate their rites at night, and in retired and obscure spots; and for this purpose no places were better fitted than the subterranean caves and passages known ever since as the Catacombs. There they met to worship, there they baptized their children and neophytes; and in many instances they deposited their dead in excavations made in the sides of these numerous galleries and avenues. These excavations were originally begun, and must have been carried on to a great extent for the purpose of procuring building materials. How far they were increased by the primitive Christians in Rome, is a matter of doubt. The length of these subterranean streets, in different directions, and taken altogether, has been estimated by late investigators at about nine hundred miles. According to Father Marchi, the Roman Catacombs may be believed to contain the prodigious number of nearly seven millions of graves. When Christianity came to be tolerated so as to admit of freedom of worship in the open day, grants of pieces of ground for the burial of the dead were made by converted publicans and Roman leaders, and thus were begun the intra-mural cemeteries, with their chapels, which, in process of time, became parish churches. Some of the cemeteries of the rural parishes were after a time comprised in the limits of the city by its subsequent extension. The history of the quarries in the tufa hills, near Naples, is similar to those of Rome: both of them supplied building materials, and both were converted into catacombs for Christian worship and burial. In the first centuries after the Christian era, so far was interment in churches from being allowed, that the presence of a solitary tomb was deemed to be sufficient cause for preventing the erection of a house of worship. The cemeteries, however, were soon placed, probably by the terms of their original grants, under ecclesiastical jurisdiction, and continued to be so during the middle ages, and as low down as the middle of the sixteenth century. It was owing to this circumstance that sanitary reforms, which seemed to be of a purly mundane valve, were so slow in being brought about. In modern times, the subject of the control of cemeteries is properly viewed as a municipal affair, and as such it ought to be studied and regulated with an eye solely to the public good.

It is not necessary to enlarge on the terrible penalties which result from a neglect of the natural laws, established on an unchangeable basis, by the Deity himself, nor to present in detail the loss of life, and in other respects wide-spread injury to the public health, caused by an infraction of these laws in the long-continued custom of interments in churches and in grave-yards within city limits. Medical men have never ceased to protest against it, and to point out the evils, sometimes amounting to frightful catastrophes, from its continuance. In some instances these results were caused by the escape of pestiferous air from recently-opened vaults in churches; in others by its extrication on a larger scale, and with more concentrated virulence, from the earth of old burying-grounds, which had been turned up with a view to their being occupied for other purposes. The efforts of Navier to enlighten the people of the government of France on the subject were so far successful, that a royal decree was issued in the following year (1776) limiting the privilege of sepulture in churches to some of the higher dignitaries in church and state. In a small tract written a few years (in 1768) before this time, the author anticipated many of the views and suggestions put forward of late years by Mr. Chadwick. Vicq d'Azyr ten years later, yielding to the solicitations of his friend D'Alembert, snatched time from his profound studies and experimental observations in anatomy and physiology, to translate a volume from the Italian of Scipio Patioli, on the subject of the selection of proper places for interment, and the dangers resulting from a neglect of the observances required on the occasion

Within the last few years the attention of the people of Great Britain has been thoroughly aroused to the enormities of intramural interments, especially as witnessed in London, by the labors of Walker and Chadwick. One cannot read without feelings of sickening and disgust, the details of the state of some of the grave-yards of the metropolis; and it must be a matter of surprise to every reflecting mind, that such scenes as are exhibited in the pages of these writers should have been so long tolerated by any people pretending to civilization, or possessed of ordinary sensibility and intelligence. In a report on extramural sepulture by the General Board of Health, it was stated that "there could not be less than two hundred, and probably more, burial-grounds in London, situated at various distances from each other, and each differing in extent. These constitute two hundred centres of more or less pollution, each pouring out unceasingly, day and night, its respective contribution of decaying matter, but the whole together, reckoning only the gas from decomposing human remains, amounting, as we have seen, in one year, to upwards of two million and a half of cubic feet. Whatever portion of these gases is not absorbed by the earth—earth already surcharged with the accumulation of centuries—and whatever part does not mix with and contaminate the water, must be emitted into the atmosphere, bearing with them, as we know, putrescent matters perceptible to sense. That these emanations do act injuriously on the health of the people resident in the immediate neighborhood of the places from which they issue, appears to us, by the evidence that has been adduced, to be indubitably established. From the law of diffusion of gases, they must be rapidly spread through the whole of the atmosphere that surrounds the metropolis, and though they thereby become diluted, and are thus rendered proportionally innocuous, yet that they do materially contribute to the contamination of the air breathed by two millions of the people, cannot, we think, admit of reasonable doubt. We submit, therefore, that a case is made out for the total prohibition of interments within the metropolis, on account of the injury resulting from the practice to public health." The argument of the General Board of Health was a convincing one, and it led to the Interment Act of 1850, the passage of which was probably facilitated by the favoring influence of the clergy of the Established Church, headed by the Bishop of London. Evidence was adduced by the Board of Health, to show that severe complaints in the vicinity of some of the church-yards, almost invariably prove fatal; and also, that the pestilential atmosphere thus formed became a fit radius for the poison of cholera during the fatal year of 1849.

But the exhalations into the atmosphere are not the only evils. Mr. George A. Walker had shown, years before, that the fluid portions of the decomposing body pass into the earth, and together with resulting gases, percolate through the walls of houses and drains, and find their way into gully-holes, and thence into the air of the streets. It is not improbable that legislative action was quickened (in the case of the Interment Act) by the annoyance to which the members of the House of Commons were exposed from a stench exhaling from gully-holes in the neighborhood. M. Gallo, the surveyor, declared it to be produced by the percolation of gases and animal compounds from the over-charged church-yard of St. Margaret's, immediately opposite. Mr. Walker, in a letter to the "editor of the *Journal of Public Health*," in which he had stated this fact, writes, in addition: "I have frequently demonstrated that a *single inspiration* of the products of human putrefaction has, in innumerable individual and collective instances, instantly destroyed life; in others produced lingering consumption, typhus, scarlet fever, &c., &c., whilst in other cases ruined health and crippled usefulness have been the clearly traceable consequences resulting from exposure to human remains in a state of decomposition." A case related by Mr. Chadwick, and which came under his own observation, may be related here, as serving to point the moral of a longer history in the same vein. In one of his walks with Professor Owen, he met with a butcher, who, in reply to some inquiries about his health, stated the following particulars. This man had lived a long time in Bear yard, near Claro market, where he was exposed to two deleterious influences—shambles on one side and a tripe-house on the other. His attention to his own impaired health, under such circumstances, was quickened by observing that it was impossible for him to keep birds, of which he was extremely fond, in this place. "You may hang up a cage," said he, "in any window of the corn-houses round Bear yard, and not a bird will live out the week." What most annoyed them among the congregation of odors, was the vapor rising from the fat in the process of preparing the tripe. Some time before this, he had occupied a room in Portugal street, overlooking a crowded church-yard, from which he often saw a dense vapor rise, that had a very offensive odor. The butcher's birds died there in brief time, and the good man found that he could only preserve new purchases by removing his quarters to Vere street, beyond the range of deleterious emanations.

Among the many wise laws enacted for the benefit of the people by the government of the republic, after the subversion of the monarchy in France, were those relating to interments. By a decree of the 23d prairial, in the year XII. of the Republic (12th June, 1804), burial in churches, temples, synagogues, and all other edifices devoted to religious worship, or in the limits of any city, town, or village, was prohibited; and, at the same time, provision was directed to be made for interring the dead in cemeteries beyond town limits. It was decreed in 1808, under the empire, that there should be no dwelling built, or well dug, within 125 yards of the new cemeteries. In Prussia, the distance of cemeteries from towns varies from 100 to 1000 yards. Some English writers recommend an interval of six to seven hundred yards between the two. The French law requires that five years must elapse before the same grave can be opened for a second interment, so that time may be allowed for the decomposition of the body first inserted, before another is deposited in its place. In the case of the city of Marseilles, with a population of one hundred thousand inhabitants, and an annual mortality of three thousand persons, it has been estimated that six thousand square metres, or about six thousand five hundred square yards of ground, would be required for the purpose of interment during a single year; assuming that to each body, separately, to be buried, there ought to be allowed a space of two square metres, or six and a half square feet. But as five years must elapse between successive interments in the same spot, the entire extent of ground necessary for the burial wants of a population of one hundred thousand persons, is thirty thousand square metres, or about thirty-two thousand five hundred square yards. Various estimates have been made of the time that must elapse before the entire decomposition and destruction of the body, leaving only the skeleton or the bones entire. Some, like Gmelin, make the period thirty to forty years; others, with Walker, at seven years; Orfila, again, found, by actual experiments instituted for the purpose, that a body, even when inclosed in a coffin, would, after interment, be reduced to the state of a skeleton in a period varying from fourteen to eighteen months. Much, in all these calculations, must depend on the nature of the soil in which interments take place. The legislation on the subject of the time that should intervene between the deposit of dead bodies in the same grave also varies. In Hesse Darmstadt, and in Prussia, an interval of thirty years is exacted; in the city of Leipsic, fifteen years; in Milan, ten years; in Munich, the capital of Bavaria, nine years. The law in France, as above stated, may be considered as meeting the exigencies of the case. Much less difference occurs in the enactments prescribing the depth of the grave opened for the reception of a dead body. In most countries, including Russia, this is somewhat more than six feet; in Frankfort on the Main, it is four feet seven inches; and in Lindon, the bishop used to direct a depth of between four and five feet.

Danger to the public health does not end with the permanent closure of a cemetery, and by the discontinuance of burial within its limits. Years must elapse before the soil can be broken up for other purposes, such as the construction of houses or the digging out of trenches or drains. It has been found that the soil of a burying-ground, in which a succession of bodies in large numbers has been laid, becomes in process of time, unfitted to bring about the putrefactive changes in bodies of more recent deposit, so as to render them, in a great degree, innocuous. The soil, under such circumstances, becomes saturated, to adopt language of recent introduction, as applied to this subject, and animalized to such a degree, that it cannot be disturbed without exhaling poisonous vapors and gases, which, in many instances, have proved suddenly fatal to those who inhaled them. Vicq d'Azyr tells of the breaking up of the soil of an old cemetery in the heart of the town of Riom, in Auvergne, with a design to public improvement, which was followed, soon after, by an endemic disease, that carried off a large number of the inhabitants, particularly of the poorer classes; and it was noticed that the mortality was greatest in the neighborhood of the cemetery. A similar calamity, from the same cause, had occurred six years before, in a small town called Ambert, also in Auvergne. The spot on which had stood a convent of the Daughters of St. Genevieve, at Paris, was eventually appropriated for the erection on it of several shops. All the first occupants of these new shops, and especially young persons, suffered from diseases nearly of the same kind—effects attributed, with good reason, to the exhalations from the bodies of those who had been buried in this ground. M. Tardieu, to whose work—a Dictionary of Public Hygiene,* &c.—we are indebted for the preceding details, writes, that he has heard many of the old inhabitants who occupied houses near the church of St. Severus, in Paris, say, that when the weather was mild and damp, there arose from the ground, which had been used for so many centuries as a place of interment, a dense vapor, of such a sickening nature as to force them to close the windows, in order to escape serious consequences. Another incident to the same purport, which occurred also in Paris, is worthy of notice. After the memorable three days of July, 1830, great difficulty was experienced in procuring immediate sepulture for those who had fallen in the fight. A provisional inhumation of a certain number was directed to take place in the ground of the Market

* Dictionnaire d'Hygiene Publique et de Salubrité. 8 vols. Paris, 1854.

of the Innocents, the spot anciently occupied as a cemetery, in long use. A trench was accordingly dug, of about twelve feet in length, by seven in width, and ten deep. When the pavement was taken up, and a layer of sand of about six inches in depth removed, a dark and greasy earth was exposed to view, mixed with bones and remains of coffins, which it was necessary to break up. The exhalations arising, in consequence, were so fetid and poisonous as to suffocate immediately one of the workmen.

Taking into consideration the alarming and often fatal effects following the disturbance of the soil of old cemeteries, the first republican government of France enacted as one of the clauses of the law respecting interments, of which we have previously spoken, that no cemetery after its final closure, should be appropriated to any other purpose short of a period of ten years. Grass or grain might be sown in it, and trees planted, but no deep digging, or foundation for buildings should be begun, until permission was regularly granted for the purpose. Reference being had to the different opinions held respecting the time required for the entire decomposition of a body after its inhumation, it may be readily supposed that there would be corresponding differences in the legislative enactments in different countries, in regard to the period that ought to elapse before a cemetery, finally closed, could be used for any other than its original purpose.

If we appeal to chemistry for aid in detecting the *deleterious gases* given out from grave-yards, and more particularly from the soil after it has been dug, as in opening a grave, or from vaults in which the dead had been deposited, we learn that the gas most largely extricated is carbonic acid, and also carbonate and sulphydrate of ammonia. Dr. Reid states, that in some church-yards he has "noticed the ground to be absolutely saturated with carbonic acid gas, so that whenever a deep grave was dug, it was filled in some hours afterwards with such an amount of carbonic acid gas, that the workmen could not descend without danger. Deaths have, indeed, occurred in some church-yards from this cause." But chemistry still fails to enlighten us fully respecting the nature or composition of those subtle poisons called miasms, which under so many circumstances generate wide-spreading and fatal disease. The vitiation of the air of the hospitals, dormitories in barracks, and in crowded assemblies, is, to a certain extent, made explicable by a minute increase of carbonic acid in these places. As evincing the great penetrativeness of these miasms, Dr. Reid tells us that he has detected their escape from graves more than twenty feet deep.

The extent of the facts now collected respecting the evils attending the practice of interments in cities in different parts of the world, and the almost uniform course of legislation, both civil and canonical, prohibiting the practice, can hardly fail of being applicable to the actual condition of things in our own country. Looking at the large and increasing population of our chief cities, the dearness of ground, and the economy of building-space, now so carefully studied, every question relating to the public health becomes of more and more importance. All preventable causes which diminish the purity of the air, or vitiate it by the addition of deleterious gases and miasms, ought to be, as far as possible, withdrawn. The increase of rural or suburban cemeteries for the burial of the dead, has doubtless had a share in abating the mischief which universal experience shows to be the frequently incidental, if not constant effect of interments in its more crowded districts. It is desirable now to take a farther and final step, and to ask that the growing partiality for extra-urban cemeteries should become not only a common, but a universal custom, sustained and enforced by formal municipal enactment.

Several years since, the Sanitary Committee of the Board of Health of Philadelphia, made a report on this subject, and offered a resolution, that in the opinion of the Board, interments of the dead within the densely populated parts of the city of Philadelphia and adjoining districts, ought to be discouraged. A carefully drawn bill, accompanying the resolutions of the Board, was sent to Harrisburgh for legislative action, but without effect. The period which has intervened between that and the present time has not diminished the evils complained of, nor rendered a reform less necessary; for the relief afforded by the voluntary extra-urban interments has not kept pace with the increase of population. The following language of the Sanitary Committee, just referred to, is as full of warning and monition to other cities as it is to the people and the municipal authorities of Philadelphia: "Your Committee are convinced that the grounds of our own metropolis are even now sources of danger to the health of our citizens, and that every year the danger resulting from these must augment. Scattered as they are over every neighborhood, surrounded by a dense and constantly-increasing population, and many of them already comparatively crowded with dead bodies, which are carelessly, and in many instances superficially interred, some of the grounds, particularly those belonging to the colored congregations, are, even now, decided nuisances, injurious to the health of the neighborhood in which they are located." Dr. Wilson Jewell, who has given much attention to public hygiene, does not hesitate to declare, after careful personal inspection and inquiry, that there is not a burial-ground in the thickly populated parts of Philadelphia, which has been in use during a period of fifteen to twenty years, which does not contain twice the number of bodies that the ground is capable of allowing to be decomposed; in other words, that it has passed its point of saturation. In some cemeteries in this city, it is no common thing to deposit three, four, and even five, bodies in one grave, until their decomposing remains reach within eighteen inches, and even a foot, of the surface.

There are grave-yards in the city, of modern date, which already show marks of being crowded with the dead; and although when first opened, they were on the borders of the city, and almost rural, they are now surrounded by streets, regularly built, which, ere many years have passed, will become densely inhabited. One of the cemeteries thus situated, and the first we believe laid out as a private speculation, a little more than thirty years ago, has received during this period, as Dr. Jewell was informed, upwards of 11,000 bodies. It occupies a space equal to one of our Philadelphia squares. Mr. White, some years ago City Inspector of New York, in his report for 1850, speaks pointedly of the nuisances of many of the grave-yards of that city. He had some of them closed during the prevalence of the Cholera in 1849. Under such circumstances, a sudden addition to the number of interments in these places, as in times of epidemic diseases, would not be without danger, and might give rise to catastrophes on a large scale, analogous to those which occurred in foreign lands, and some of which have been recorded in the present report.

Not having been required to invesigate the whole subject of interments, we do not deem it necessary to specify the kinds of soil most favorable for the purpose of accelerating the desired changes in the decomposition of the body buried, nor have we inquired into the sanitary influence of plantations of trees in cemeteries, with a view to the purification of the air of these spots. We must not omit, however, referring to a plan recently suggested, and in some places carried into effect, in England. It is, to surround the bodies of the dead, before they are finally inclosed, with a layer some four inches thick of finely powdered *wood or peat charcoal.* By this means the decay of the animal textures would go on rapidly, and without giving rise to dangerous exhalations. In the burial of the poor this plan merits a favorable consideration, and it must indeed commend itself as worthy of adoption by all classes. The experiments of Dr. Stenhouse place the subject of the operation of vegetable charcoal on dead bodies in a new and instructive light, by showing, contrary to popular belief, that, although a deodorizing and disinfecting agent, it is not an antiseptic proper, which gives stability to organic matter, and prevents its decomposition. Charcoal, and, in less degree, clay, produce a species of slow combustion, by which the miasms are gradually consumed.

Without being called upon to look at the subject of intramural interments under its purely moral and religious aspects, we are nevertheless free to allude to the depressing, and in such times morbid influence, exerted on the community by its being compelled to witness the frequent, and in visitations of certain fearful epidemics, the almost continual succession of funeral processions. This is a matter of public health, in discussing which, medical testimony cannot be overlooked. Were it necessary, clerical experience could also be invoked in favor of suburban burials in preference to those in the city, whether regard be had to the desirableness of the uninterrupted solemnities of the burial service, the avoidance of whatever would grate on the already harrowed feelings of attending relatives and friends, and the preserving unbroken the associations of an elevated and religious character, with the sight of the memorials to the dead and of the spot where their bodies rest. * * * *

There are yet other matters worthy of notice which might serve to show still further the importance and economy of sanitary measures to cities, and of which it would be desirable to treat. A topic of considerable moment in all commercial cities is the structure of the wharves, so that there shall be nothing in the materials of which they are made, susceptible of decay and decomposition. So also of quays in every town on the banks of a river, and their construction so as to narrow the channel and diminish the exposed surface at low water on both of the sides of the river. One measure in the internal hygiene of cities ought to be a careful supervision of all stables, cow-houses, and piggeries, and vigilance in the removal of heaps of manure, accumulated under no matter what excuse. Ascending the scale of the duties of sanitary supervision, would come that of manufactories and of work-shops, which may be termed public, by their extent and the number of persons employed; also of all buildings in which people assemble in numbers at stated times. Minute inquiries are made into the structure and arrangement of the rooms, and the number and plan of fire-places, furnaces, and stoves, before an insurance against fire can be effected. Why then should there be any hesitation about a similarly careful investigation by the sanitary authorities, with a view to insurance against preventable diseases among the inmates of a house?

In concluding this report, its author must express his regret at not having had the time to treat in a rigidly methodical manner the various topics which have come under notice. He submits, however, that, while adhering with some closeness to the terms of his instructions, he has made out a case showing the paramount necessity for a methodical and liberal, yet prudent, system of sanitary legislation, and the wisdom of adopting such a code as the Metropolitan Sanitary one, which will be presented to the Convention by one of our Committee. The time, we may hope, is not remote when the writer on sanitary subjects, especially if he desires exactness of detail, and comparisons and results of an authentic kind, set forth numerically, will not be obliged, as he now is, to procure most of his arguments and enforcements of reform from abroad, owing to the deficiency of statistical knowledge and the underrating its value here at home, so that he is deprived of the requisite data either to show with accuracy the extent of existing evils, or to point out the means for their removal. One measure of the highest importance, and without which nothing trustworthy can be learned of vital statistics, direct or comparative, is a system of births, deaths, and marriages, regularly carried out in every State of the Union.

DRAFT

OF A

SANITARY CODE FOR CITIES,

(Reported to the Committee on Internal Hygiene.)

BY HENRY G. CLARK, M.D., OF BOSTON,

ONE OF THE COMMITTEE.

CONTENTS.

DRAFT

OF AN ACT FOR ESTABLISHING GENERAL AND LOCAL BOARDS OF HEALTH, AND FOR OTHER SANITARY PURPOSES.*

AN ACT, *in addition to existing Acts, for promoting the Public Health.*

WHEREAS it is expedient that further and more effectual provision should be made for improving the sanitary condition of populous places: Be it therefore enacted by the Senate and House of Representatives in General Court assembled, and by the authority of the same, as follows; that is to say:

I. This act may be cited for all purposes as "The Public Health Act, 1860."

II. The Governor of the Commonwealth, with the advice and consent of the Council, shall appoint five discreet and suitable persons, three at least of whom shall be Doctors of Medicine, who, together with the Secretary of State for the time being, and the Governor, ex-officiis, shall together be and constitute a Board, to be called "The General Board of Health;" and shall have and execute all the powers and duties necessary for superintending and promoting the general sanitary affairs of the State.

III. They shall hold their offices for five years, or until others are appointed in their place; and they shall be sworn to the faithful performance of their duty.

IV. They shall meet at such convenient times as they deem expedient, and their necessary official expenses shall be paid out of the Treasury of the State; but they shall receive no other compensation for their services.

V. They shall appoint a competent person, who may also be the Register-General, to be the Secretary or Actuary of

* For the debate on this Report, see pp. 86, *et seq.*, and pp. 226, *et seq.*, of the Proceedings.

the Board, who shall receive such a salary, not exceeding dollars per annum, as the Board shall determine. They shall also appoint, if need be, a competent physician, who shall be styled a Medical Health Officer, and another competent person for Surveyor, who shall be removable at their pleasure, and who shall receive such fees or other compensation as the Board may, from time to time, determine.

They may also appoint and employ such other persons as may be necessary to carry into effect the sanitary laws of the State, and delegate to them the necessary powers, subject to the approval of the local Boards of Health, hereinafter provided for.

VI. They shall consider and decide upon sanitary questions submitted to them by the State, cities, towns, or local Boards of Health.

VII. They shall, by reports or otherwise, diffuse information to the inhabitants of the State on sanitary matters; and shall aid, by regulations, suggestions, and by furnishing blanks, &c., the various local Boards of Health.

VIII. The corporate authorities of the various cities and towns of this Commonwealth are hereby authorized and empowered to establish local Boards of Health, and to enact and enforce, generally and severally, such laws, ordinances, and regulations, as they may deem expedient or necessary for promoting the sanitary condition of the said cities and towns, and as are not inconsistent with the Constitution and laws of the State.

IX. And the said authorities are also authorized to delegate to the said local Boards of Health, or other agents, all the powers necessary for the convenient execution of said laws, ordinances, and regulations.

X. All acts, and parts of acts, incompatible with this act, are hereby repealed.

DRAFT

OF AN ORDINANCE FOR PROMOTING THE HEALTH OF TOWNS.

SANITARY CODE FOR CITIES.

Whereas, by an Act of the Legislature, in the year 1860, *entitled "The Public Health Act," this Corporation has been duly authorized and empowered to make all needful rules and regulations for the preservation of the health of its inhabitants: Be it therefore ordained by the Councils of the Town of——, and by authority thereof, as follows, to wit:*

I. This Ordinance shall be cited for all purposes as "The Sanitary Code for Cities."

II. The duty of executing and enforcing the provisions of this "Code" is hereby vested in a Board of Health, at least one-third of the members of which shall be Doctors of Medicine, to be chosen by the Councils, or in such other way as the legal voters may determine; and they are hereby constituted the local Board of Health, with all the powers and privileges usually invested in Boards of Health, and with such further especial powers as may be conferred by the provisions of this Ordinance.

III. And said local Board, or its authorized agents, shall have the right at all times to enter into or upon any premises for the purposes of this Ordinance, and also to call upon any of the officers or of the police, to aid them in the execution of its provisions.

IV. In the construction, and for the purposes of this Ordinance, the following words and expressions shall have the meanings hereinafter assigned to them; that is to say:

The term "person," and words applying to any individual, shall apply to, and include corporations, aggregate or sole.

The term "owner" shall mean the person for the time being entitled to the rent of the land or premises in connection with which the term is used, whether on his own account, or as trustee or agent for any other person.

The expression, "Improvement Commissioners," shall mean the commissioners, trustees, or other persons, intrusted by any local act with powers of cleansing, paving, or otherwise improving any town.

The term "town" shall also include "cities," or any other municipal corporation.

The term "land" shall include messuages, buildings, lands, and hereditaments of every tenure; also rivers, streams, wells, and waters of every description; also easements of any description in respect of the foregoing particulars.

The term "waste-pipe" shall mean the pipe which discharges the waste-water from within any house into the drain.

The term "drain" shall mean any drain of, and used for the drainage of one building only, or premises within the same curtilage, and made merely for the purpose of communicating therefrom with a cess-pool or other like receptacle for drainage, or with a sewer, into which the drainage, of two or more buildings or premises, occupied by different persons, is conveyed.

The term "sewer" shall mean and include sewers and drains of every description, except drains to which the word "drain," interpreted as aforesaid, applies.

The term, "slaughter-house," shall mean and include the buildings and places commonly called slaughter-houses and knackers' yards, and any building or place used for slaughtering cattle, horses, or animals of any description.

The term "district" shall mean the entire area, places, or parts of places, comprised within the limits of any district to which this "Code," or any part thereof, shall be applied.

The term "street" shall include a square, circus, crescent, terrace, place, row, mews, alley, court, passage, or or other like place in which the houses are continuous, or separated only by small intervals of space.

The word "house" shall include schools, factories, and other buildings, in which more than twenty persons are assembled at one time.

SANITARY SURVEY.

V. There shall be made, annually, a thorough sanitary survey of the town or district, as the case may be; and at any other time, when it shall appear from the returns to the Registrar that the number of deaths shall exceed, annually, that of twenty-five to a thousand of the population of such place.

And the Board of Health may, if in their discretion they think fit, direct the Medical Health Officer to cause public inquiry to be made as to the following matters and things, or any of them; that is to say:

As to the sewerage, drainage, and water-supply;

As to the number and sanitary condition of the inhabitants;

As to the accumulation of filth;

As to any other matter of which the Board may require to be informed.

VI. The said survey shall be made in the manner following, to wit:

The Medical Health Officer shall have the right to call upon the Chief of Police, who shall detail for this service a sufficient number of the regular patrol force, who shall act as inspecting health officers. But during an epidemic season, or when any medical facts are to be obtained, the inspectors shall be Doctors or Students of Medicine.

Upon receiving his instructions, each officer will commence and diligently prosecute his inquiries; carefully noticing the state of the streets, lanes, courts, passages, common stairs, houses, rooms, cellars, yards, or vacant lots in his assigned district; reporting in detail, and in writing, all accumulations of filth; all cases where the waste-pipes, drains, or water-closets are foul or obstructed; all cases of prevailing sickness, especially where there is great overcrowding, or unusual destitution; also all cases of dead bodies found in single-living rooms.

The reports may be made in the manner of the blank forms hereto annexed. (See Appendix A.)

VII. When any nuisance or other source of disease is discovered, notice, in the proper form (see Appendix B), is to be served upon the owners or occupants, forthwith to abate the same, and in case of refusal or neglect for a period of   hours, the Medical Health Officer is authorized and directed to cause the same to be abated or removed in the most summary manner; and he is hereby authorized to call upon the Chief of Police, the Engineer, the Registrar, and the Superintendents of Health, of Streets, and of Drains, to aid him in such removal.

The expense of such removals or abatements of nuisances (of which an accurate account is to be kept), shall be chargeable to the owners or occupants of the premises.

These measures shall be so continuously pursued as to prevent, as far as possible, any reaccumulation of the causes of disease sought to be removed, and each officer shall be held strictly responsible for the sanitary condition of his assigned district.

All persons, acting under and by the authority of this order, may be authorized to enter upon and into any premises which it may be necessary to visit, in compliance with its provisions; but their object in so doing must be first stated to the occupants, and all unnecessary annoyance to them most carefully avoided.

SEWERAGE.

VIII. The said Board of Health may, if they shall think fit, cause to be prepared, or procure a map, exhibiting a system of sewerage for effectually draining their district for the purpose of this Ordinance, upon a scale to be prescribed by the General Board of Health; and every such map shall be kept at the office of the said Board, and shall, at all reasonable times, be open to the inspection of the tax-payers of the district to which it applies.

IX. All sewers, drains, or waste-pipes, whether at present existing, or which shall be hereafter constructed, shall be entirely under the management and control of the Board of Health.

X. The Board of Health shall cause their district to be effectually drained upon the plan recommended by the General Board of Health of Great Britain; and they shall have power within such district from time to time to do any of the following things:

(1.) To repair, arch over, enlarge, lessen, or otherwise alter, any existing sewer or drain.

(2.) To construct any new sewer or drain, with a like power of repairing and altering the same.

(3.) To discontinue, close up, or destroy any sewer or drain.

(4.) To carry any sewer, drain, or pipe, for the distribution of sewage, through, across, or under any turnpike or other road, or county bridge, or any street, or place laid out as, or intended for a street, or under any cellar or vault which may be under the pavement or carriage-way of any street or intended street, upon condition of making good all damage done by them; or if it is deemed necessary by the Surveyor of the Board, into, under, or through any lands whatever, upon making due compensation for the same:

Subject, nevertheless, to the restrictions hereinafter mentioned; that is to say:

(1.) All waste-pipes, sewers, and drains shall be so constructed and kept as not to create a nuisance, or be injurious to health.

(2.) If, by the exercise of any of the above powers, any person is deprived of the lawful use of any sewer or drain, the Board shall provide for his use some other sewer or drain equally convenient.

XI. The Board of Health are hereby empowered, upon making due compensation, to do the following things; that is to say:

(1.) To construct, either above or under ground, such reservoirs and other works as may be necessary for holding the sewage flowing from the sewers of their district, or to provide outfalls for the same.

(2.) To cause the sewers to empty into such reservoirs or outfalls, by means of connecting sewers, or such other means as they think fit.

(3.) To contract with any company or person for the sale of such sewage, or for the distribution of it over any land; and any such company for these purposes shall have the same privileges, and be subject to the same conditions, as would the local Board.

(4.) To contract for, purchase, or take on lease any buildings, engines, materials, or apparatus for the purpose of receiving, storing, disinfecting, or distributing any such sewage, and to lease or assign such buildings, engines, materials, or apparatus to any company or person with whom the said Board of Health may contract as aforesaid.

(5.) To purchase or take on lease any land where such purchase or leasing is necessary for carrying into execution the above objects.

XII. No person shall, without the consent of the Board of Health, do the following things, or any of them:

(1.) Cause any waste-pipe, sewer, or drain, to communicate with, or be emptied into any sewer of the Board of Health.

(2.) Cause any vault, arch, or cellar, to be newly built or constructed under any public street; and if any sewer, drain, vault, arch, or cellar is made, in contravention of this Ordinance, the Board of Health may cause the same to be pulled down, if they shall think fit, and the expenses incurred by them in so doing shall be repaid to them by the offender, and be recoverable from him in a summary manner.

XIII. Any owner or occupier of premises adjoining any district, may, with the consent of the Board of Health, cause any sewer or drain from such premises to communicate with any sewer of the Board, upon such conditions as they shall mutually agree.

XIV. Whenever it appears to the Board of Health that any house or other building, already built, is without any waste-pipe, drain, or water-closet, or that they do not empty into such place as is efficient for effectual drainage, the Board may by notice require the owner of such house or building, within a reasonable time therein specified, to make a sufficient drain, of a construction approved by the Board of Health, emptying as follows: that is to say, if the sea, or a sewer of the Board of Health, or any sewer which they are entitled to use, is within one hundred feet of the site of such house or dwelling, emptying, as the Board may direct, either into the sea or such sewer; but if no such means of drainage are within that distance, then emptying into such covered cess-pool, or other place, not being under any house, and not being within such distance from any house, as the Board of Health direct; and if the person, on whom such notice is served, fail to comply with the same, the Board may themselves do the work required, and assess the expenses to the owner or occupant aforesaid.

XV. The following rules shall be observed with regard to drains of houses not already built:

(1.) The drains of every such new house or building as aforesaid, shall be covered in, and be of such size and materials, at such level, and with such fall, as may be effectual, in the opinion of the Surveyor or Engineer of the Board, to secure a proper drainage of such house or building, and its appurtenances.

(2.) If the sea, or a sewer of the Board of Health, or a sewer which they are entitled to use, is within one hundred feet of any part of the site of such new house or building, the drains so to be constructed shall communicate with such one of those means of drainage as the Board direct.

(3.) If no such means of drainage are within that distance, then the last-mentioned drains shall communicate with, and be emptied into such covered cess-pool or other place, not being under any house, and not being within such distance from any house, as the Board of Health direct.

(4.) The Board shall have the power of enforcing and directing the construction of "dry privies," vaults, or cess-pools, wherever the nature of the ground, the building materials in use, the imperfect supply of water, or any other circumstances, shall render this necessary for the public health, especially for the preservation of the purity of streams, springs, or other sources of fresh water.

But: *a.* These privies or vaults shall be so constructed that their contents can be periodically, conveniently, and safely removed for agricultural or other purposes. *b.* And they shall be effectually deodorized by some proper and sufficient drying or deodorizing agent, so that they will not be dangerous or offensive, either while undisturbed or during the process of removal.

(5.) Any house or building which, during the process of repairs, shall be pulled down to the ground floor, shall be subject to the same regulations as if it were a new house or building.

XVI. If any house or building is built or re-built, or any drain or vault constructed contrary to the foregoing provisions, the owner of such house or building shall be subject to the following liabilities; that is to say:

(1.) He shall incur such a penalty for each offense as the Board may determine; or,

(2.) The Board of Health, after due notice, and his failure to comply therewith, may thereupon proceed to do the work required, and assess the expenses upon said owner.

CLEANSING.

XVII. The following works shall be done in respect to scavenging:

(1.) All public streets, together with the foot-pavements thereof, shall be properly cleansed and watered; all roads shall be properly cleansed, and the whole or any part of such roads may, in the discretion of the Board of Health, be watered.

(2.) All dust, ashes, and rubbish shall be carried away from the premises of the inhabitants.

(3.) All privies and cess-pools shall be, from time to time, emptied and cleansed; but their contents shall first be deodorized. And the Board of Health may themselves undertake, or contract with any person to undertake the aforesaid works, or any of them.

XVIII. No person, except by direct authority of the Board, shall undertake to remove any of the substances mentioned in the preceding section, or obstruct the Board or its agents in so doing.

XIX. In cases where the Board of Health do not themselves undertake, or contract with any person to undertake, the works heretofore named, they may make by-laws imposing on the occupier of any premises any or all of the duties of cleansing. They may affix reasonable penalties for the breach of said by-laws.

XX. Whenever the Board of Health shall be satisfied that the number of persons occupying any tenement or building is so great as to be the cause of nuisance, or sickness, or a source of filth; or that any tenements or buildings are not furnished with vaults constructed according to the provisions of this Ordinance; or with a sufficient number of privies or water-closets, with underground drains; with proper ash-pits, or with a proper water-supply; or that, from any cause, they are in a condition which is prejudicial or dangerous to the public health, or to the health of the occupants themselves—they may thereupon issue notice in writing to such persons, or any of them—that is to say, the owner, agent, or occupant, or either of them—to cause either or all of these deficiencies to be supplied, and the premises put into a cleanly and proper condition, within such reasonable time as they shall appoint; and in case of neglect or refusal to obey such notice, they may themselves cause the alterations and cleansings to be done forthwith, and the expense of it shall be paid by such owner, agent, occupant, or other person. Or they may, if they think fit, issue notice to the persons inhabiting such tenement, or to the owner or agent, requiring them to remove from, and quit the premises, within such time as the Board may deem reasonable; and if the person or persons so notified, or any of them, shall neglect or refuse to remove from said tenement or building, the Board of Health are hereby fully authorized and empowered thereupon forcibly to remove the same.

XXI. The Board of Health may make and issue by-laws for the prevention of nuisances arising from filth, dust, ashes, and rubbish, or from the keeping of animals, and may annex reasonable penalties for the breach of said by-laws.

XXII. The business of a blood-boiler, bone-boiler, bone-burner, fell-monger, slaughterer of animals of any description not fit for human food, soap-boiler, tallow-melter, tripe-boiler, or other noxious or offensive business, trade or manufacture, shall not, without the consent of the Board, be established within the district; and the Board may make such regulations in regard to these occupations as they may deem expedient.

XXIII. When the contents of any sewer, or any accumulations of filth, are discharged into any river or stream, in the bed of which the quantity of water is so much diminished, either by drought during the summer, or by any other cause, as to be insufficient to keep the channel clear, the Board of Health may, by excavations or other operations, so deepen the channel as that the flow of water will be accelerated, and the contents of said sewers or drains be thereby prevented from accumulating and stagnating in parts thereof, to the injury of the health, and the annoyance of the surrounding population.

XXIV. No person, without the license of the Board of Health, shall throw into, or leave in, or upon any street, square, or vacant lot, or into any pond or body of water, within the limits of this town or district, any dead animal, dirt, saw-dust, soot, ashes, cinders, shavings, hair, manure, oyster, clam, or lobster shells, waste water, rubbish, or filth of any kind, or any refuse, animal, or vegetable whatsoever. Nor shall any person throw into, or leave in or upon any dock, flats, or tide-water, within the jurisdiction of this district, any dead animal or other foul or offensive matter, except as above provided.

XXV. The owners and occupants of livery and other stables, within the limits of the town or district, as the case may be, shall not wash or clean their carriages or horses, or cause them to be washed or cleaned, in the streets, nor otherwise encumber the same; they shall keep their stables and yards clean, and shall not permit more than four cart-loads of manure to accumulate in or near the same, at any one time between the first day of May and the first day of November; nor within that period suffer the same to be removed, except between the hour of twelve at night and two hours after sunrise.

XXVI. Swine shall not be kept within the limits of the town without a permit from the Board of Health.

SLAUGHTER-HOUSES.

XXVII. No place shall be used or occupied as a slaughter-house except by permission of the Board of Health; and they may make by-laws with respect to their management, and for keeping the same in a wholesome state.

THE MARKETS.

XXVIII. The Medical Health Officer, or either of the Inspectors or Agents of the Board of Health, may, at all reasonable times, enter into and inspect any shop, building, stall, or place kept or used for the sale of butchers' meat, poultry, or fish, or as a slaughter-house; and to examine any animal, carcass, meat, poultry, game, flesh, or fish, which may be therein; and in case either of them, being intended for the food of man, shall appear to be unfit for such food, the same may be seized; and if it prove to be unwholesome, he shall order the same to be destroyed, or be so disposed of as to prevent its being again exposed for sale.

XXIX. No person shall be permitted to bring into town for sale, or sell, or offer for sale, any fresh fish, until the same shall have been cleansed of their entrails and refuse parts; and such entrails and parts shall be thrown overboard below low-water mark; and shall never be kept beyond the flowing of the next tide; and until so thrown overboard, they shall be kept in a close and safe manner on board the vessels or boats on which the fish are brought. And no person shall sell, or offer for sale, fish of any kind, unless the same be kept in covered stalls, fish-boxes, or other houses, which shall always be clean and in good order; or, in clean covered carts, or boxes, well secured from the rays of the sun.

XXX. No person shall have in his possession for sale, or shall sell, or offer for sale, within the limits of the town, any vegetables whatever, excepting green peas in the pod, and green corn in the inner husks, which have not previously been divested of such parts or appendages as are not commonly used for food.

XXXI. No person shall land on any wharf or other place, or shall bring into town, any decayed or damaged grains, vegetables, or fruit, without a permit from an officer of the Board of Health, and in such manner as he may direct.

XXXII. No person shall sell any adulterated or unwholesome food or drink; and if, upon being notified by the Board to discontinue such practice, he shall neglect or refuse to obey such order, he may be ejected from the precincts of the market, and such articles of food or drink may be seized and destroyed.

XXXIII. If any person shall falsify any milk, by adulteration with water or otherwise, or by the abstraction of its cream, or any other substance originally belonging to it; or, if any person having reason to believe it so falsified, shall sell the same, or cause it to be sold, he shall be liable to have it seized and destroyed, and to fine and imprisonment, and to have placards, stating his offense and the sentence imposed, posted up at his place of business or elsewhere, as the Board may determine. This shall also apply to milk from diseased cows.

XXXIV. All bread, except as specially provided to the contrary in this section, shall be sold by weight.

A loaf of bread shall be two pounds in weight; and bread may be baked and sold in whole, half, three-quarter and quarter loaves, but not otherwise, except in bread composed in chief part of rye or maize.

Small rolls and fancy bread, weighing less than one quarter of a pound each, may be baked and sold without regard to weight.

In every shop or place where bread is sold by retail, and in each front window thereof, there shall be conspicuously placed a card, on which shall be legibly printed a list of the different kinds and qualities of loaves sold there, with the price of each per loaf, and half, three-quarter, and quarter loaf.

All bread, except small rolls and fancy bread of less than a quarter of a pound each, sold in any shop or place, shall be weighed in the presence of the buyer, and if found deficient in weight, bread shall be added to make up the weight required by law.

Any person, who shall violate any of the provisions of this act, shall forfeit for each offense the sum of dollars, and he shall also be liable to the penalties provided in Section XXXIII.

XXXV. And the Board of Health is also hereby authorized to make, promulgate, and enforce such by-laws for the government of the market-houses and the sale of provisions as they may think expedient.

DRAM-SHOPS AND DRINKING-HOUSES.

XXXVI. All unlicensed dram-shops and drinking-houses for the sale of intoxicating drinks, are hereby declared to be nuisances, and may be abated as such, by the Board of Health.

COMMON LODGING-HOUSES.

XXXVII. No person shall keep a common lodging-house without a license from the Board of Health, after inspection by the Medical Health Officer of the Board. And a register shall be kept, in which shall be entered the name of every person applying to register any common lodging-house kept by him, and the situation of every such house; and the said Board shall, from time to time, make by-laws for fixing the number of lodgers who may be received into each house so registered; for promoting cleanliness and ventilation therein; and with respect to the inspection thereof, and the conditions and restrictions under which such inspection may be made; and the person keeping any such lodging-house shall give access to the same, when required by any person who shall produce the written authority of the Board, for the purpose of inspecting the same, or for introducing or using therein any disinfecting process; and the expenses incurred by the said Board in such process shall be assessed and collected from the keeper of said house; and if any such keeper of such lodging-house shall neglect or refuse to obey the directions of the Board of Health, he shall forfeit his license.

CELLARS.

XXXVIII. No cellar or underground room shall be let or occupied separately as a dwelling, without being registered and licensed by the Board, and unless it possess the following requisites; that is to say:

(1.) Unless the same is in every part thereof at least seven feet in height, measured from floor to ceiling thereof; nor,

(2.) Unless the same is at least one foot of its height above the surface of the street or ground adjoining, or nearest to the same; nor,

(3.) Unless there is outside of, and adjoining such cellar or room, and extending along the entire frontage thereof, and upwards, from six inches below the level of the floor thereof, up to the surface of the said street or ground, an open area of at least three feet wide in every part; nor,

(4.) Unless the same is well and effectually drained, and secured against the rise of effluvia from any sewer or drain; nor,

(5.) Unless there is appurtenant to such cellar or room the use of a water-closet or privy, as the Board may require; and of an ash-pit, furnished with proper doors and coverings; nor,

(6.) Unless the same has a fire-place, with a proper chimney, or other ventilating flue; nor,

(7.) Unless the same has an external window of at least nine superficial feet in area, clear of the sash-frame, and made to open in such manner as is approved by the Surveyor of the Board.

And whosoever lets, occupies, or continues to let, or knowingly suffers to be occupied, any cellar or underground room, contrary to this section, shall be liable to forfeit his license, and shall be subject, if he persist, to such other penalty as the Board may determine: and every cellar or underground room, in which any person passes the night, shall be deemed to be occupied as a dwelling within the meaning of this Ordinance; but the above rule shall be qualified in respect to areas as follows:

(1.) In any area adjoining a cellar or underground room, there may be placed steps necessary for access to such cellar or room, if the same are so placed as not to be over or across the said external window.

(2.) Over or across any such area there may be steps necessary for access to any building above the cellar or room to which such area adjoins, if the same be so placed as not to be over or across any such external window.

NEW STREETS AND HOUSES.

XXXIX. The Board, with the consent of the town councils, and with the advice and aid of the Engineer or Surveyor, shall fix and determine the following matters; that is to say:

(1.) With respect to the level and width of new streets, and the provisions for the sewerage and paving thereof.

(2.) With respect to the structure of walls of new buildings, in reference to stability and the prevention of fires.

(3.) With respect to the sufficiency of the space in connection with buildings, to secure a free circulation of air, and the ventilation of buildings.

(4.) With reference to the drainage of buildings, to water-closets, privies, and cess-pools in connection with buildings, and to the closing and prohibition of buildings or parts of buildings unfit for human habitation.

The regulations of this Section and of Sections XX., XXXVII., and XXXVIII, shall be considered also as particularly applicable, and may be enforced in regard to *Model Houses*, and to houses already built or occupied.

They may annex such penalties, and further provide for the observance of these regulations by such by-laws as they think necessary, and may alter or pull down any work begun or done in contravention of such by-laws: *Provided*, however, that no person shall be deprived by any by-law of such right of appeal as is hereinafter given in respect of by-laws.

SUPPLY OF WATER.

XL. The following provisions shall be observed with respect to the supply of water:

(1.) All public wells, pumps, conduits, or other works used for the gratuitous supply of water to the inhabitants shall vest in, and be under the control of, a Board of Improvement Commissioners, or such persons as may be chosen for that purpose by the town councils, with the approbation of the Board of Health, who shall have the right to direct the use of the water for any sanitary purpose.

(2.) A sufficient quantity shall be supplied for domestic purposes, the takers paying such fixed rates therefor as may be determined; and,

(3.) May be supplied to any public baths or wash-houses, or for manufacturing purposes, on such terms and conditions as may be mutually agreed upon.

(4.) A sufficient quantity shall be provided for flushing sewers and drains, for putting out fires, for cleaning and watering the streets, and for other public purposes.

(5.) The expense of providing a supply of water for the foregoing purposes, over what shall be paid by the takers, shall be assessed on the inhabitants, or paid in such other way as the councils shall determine.

XLI. Any person who willfully wastes or fouls the water, or injures any of the works for its supply, shall be liable to such penalties as the Board or the Commissioners shall determine, and shall be also liable to a suit for damage at common law.

XLII. When it shall appear that any house or tenement let to other persons than the owners thereof is not in any way supplied with water, the owners of such house or tenement shall be notified by the Board of Health to supply the same; and in case of refusal, or neglect to do so within a reasonable time, the Board may supply the same at the expense of the owner, or, at its option, vacate the premises.

VENTILATION.

XLIII. No cellar, lodging-house, or other "house," intended for the constant occupation of not less than ten persons, or for the occasional assemblage of large numbers of persons, shall be used or occupied, except under the following conditions; that is to say:

(1.) Unless the same shall be provided with some effectual ventilation, as follows:

a. By ventiducts for supplying fresh air of a suitable temperature, which shall have a capacity of not less than one hundred square inches for every twenty-five persons, and in the same proportion for any greater or less number; or,

b. By some other mode capable of supplying pure air to each person at the rate of four cubic feet per minute.

c. By discharging-ventiducts, which open directly into heated flues, or which are conducted into the outer air above the roof, and then terminated by a suitable cowl or cap, and which shall have a capacity of not less than two-thirds of that of the admitting ventiducts; or,

d. By an open fire-place; an Arnott's valve; an opening into some other ventilated apartment; or,

e. By some other effectual method of expelling the foul air.

(2.) Or unless the drains, vaults, and water-closets are securely trapped and effectually ventilated:

a. By connecting them with the rain-water spouts; or,

b. If within the house, as in the case of water-closets, by a ventilating flue opening above the roof, or which is connected with a heated flue.

PLEASURE-GROUNDS.

XLIV. The Board of Health may, with the approval of the Town Council, hold, purchase by agreement, take on lease, maintain, lay out, plant, and improve land for the purpose of being laid out as public walks or pleasure-grounds, and support or contribute towards any premises provided for such purposes by any person whomsoever.

EPIDEMIC AND CONTAGIOUS DISEASES.

XLV. When any epidemic, endemic, or contagious disease shall threaten the town, or affect any part of the same, in order that measures of precaution may be taken with promptitude, according to the exigency of the case, the Board of Health may issue such directions and regulations as they may think fit; and they shall provide for the frequent cleansing of streets and public ways, and for the cleaning, purifying, ventilating, and disinfecting of houses by the owners or agents; for the removal of nuisances; to provide for the sick by establishing and opening temporary hospitals, and for the speedy interment of the dead; and, generally, for preventing or mitigating such malignant diseases, in such manner as to the said Board seems expedient. And if any vessel, having any contagious or other malignant disease on board, or having come from ports where such diseases are prevailing, shall arrive at either of the wharves, or come to anchor near them, she shall be ordered by the Health Officer to proceed to Quarantine, there to report herself to the Quarantine Physician.

PUBLIC VACCINATION.

XLVI. In order to prevent the spread of small-pox, and to diffuse the benefits of vaccination, it is hereby ordained that there shall be provided a suitable apartment for the Medical Officer of the Board, at which place he shall attend at such times as the Board may direct; and he shall vaccinate without charge any inhabitant of this town, not previously vaccinated, who may apply for that purpose. And he shall give certificates of said vaccination, without which no child shall be admitted to the public schools. And he shall also always have on hand, as far as practicable, a sufficient quantity of vaccine lymph to supply the physicians of the public institutions.

INTERMENT OF THE DEAD.

XLVII. The Board of Health, with the consent of the councils, shall, from time to time, provide, in such places as, having regard to the public health, may appear to them expedient, and within or without the limits of the district, burial-grounds of sufficient extent for the decent interment of the bodies of all persons dying within the district; and it shall be lawful for the said Board, in case it appears to them necessary or expedient so to do, to enlarge any burial-ground provided by them under this Ordinance, and to make any road to such ground, or to enlarge or improve any existing road for facilitating the approach to such burial-ground; and for providing any such burial-ground, or improving it, they may purchase any lands which it may appear to them expedient to purchase for that purpose.

XLVIII. They may inclose and lay out the burial-grounds thus provided, and build therein suitable chapels for the performance of the burial service, and such other buildings and works as may appear to them fitting and proper.

XLIX. When the said Board shall be of opinion that interment (otherwise than in the burial-grounds provided in this Ordinance) should be discontinued, wholly, or subject to any exception or exceptions, in any part or parts of the town, they shall, after due notice, order their discontinuance; and the grounds so discontinued shall be closed or fenced up in such a manner as to protect the public health, and secure proper respect to the bodies interred therein. And this section shall also be considered as applying to vaults under churches and chapels, as well as to the open burial-grounds.

L. No burial shall take place, or be permitted in any of the so-closed grounds, or under, or in any churches or chapels to which this order shall have been applied, except in the cases following; that is to say:

(1.) In case of long previously-existing private rights of sepulture, the Board may, in their discretion, give a license, under such restrictions as may seem to them proper.

(2.) Or if, on representations properly made to them, they may deem the permission, if granted in exceptional cases, not prejudicial to the public health.

LI. But any and all persons who may have, by any such discontinuance or closure of any burial-ground, as provided for in section XLIX, been deprived of any rights of sepulture, shall have in the newly-consecrated ground the same rights as they respectively would have had in the burial-places thus closed and discontinued; or they shall be otherwise equitably compensated therefor.

LII. The relatives of any deceased person, with the consent of the Registrar, or other person having charge of the closed ground in which the body of the deceased has been interred, and subject to the regulations of the Board, may cause such body to be removed to, and re-interred in any burial-ground provided under this Ordinance.

LIII. The Board, from time to time, may make regulations as to the depth and formation of the graves and places of interment, the nature of the coffins to be received in the burial-grounds thus provided, the time and mode of removing bodies, and generally, as to all matters connected with the good order of such burial-grounds, and as to the conduct of funeral processions, and the convenient exercise of the rights of interment therein: and such regulations shall be printed and published, and shall be fixed and continued on some conspicuous part of every such burial-ground.

LIV. All burials shall be registered in books to be kept for the purpose, in the manner directed, and by the officer whose duty it shall be made by the Board of Health.

LV. No burial shall take place, except upon the written permit of the Registrar or Coroner, who, before issuing said permit, shall require to be furnished with the name, sex, age, rank, profession or occupation, and the residence at the time of death, of said person; nor shall such permit be then issued, except the cause of the death of said deceased person shall be fully certified to the Registrar or other permitting officer, by some regularly-licensed or competent physician or surgeon.

LVI. The Board may, at any time after the passage of this Ordinance, build, or otherwise provide, in suitable and convenient locations, houses for the reception and care of the bodies of the dead, previously to, and until interment, and make arrangements for the reception and care of such bodies therein, and appoint fit officers for such houses of reception; and they may also appoint or provide medical or other officers, who, in cases where the friends of the deceased so desire, may cause the body of the deceased to be decently removed to one of the houses of reception provided for under this section.

LVII. "Wakes" shall not be permitted, without the special leave, in writing, of the Board, or of its authorized agent: nor then, if the death has been occasioned by any malignant or epidemic disease; or if from any cause the health of those who would be there present, or of others with whom they would be in contact, would be thereby endangered.

LVIII. The Board may, from time to time, fix, according to a just and regular scale of charges, the rates in classes, varying according to circumstances, of prices for the conduct of funerals; but so that in respect of the lowest of such classes, the funeral may be conducted with decency and solemnity.

GENERAL PROVISIONS.

LIX. There shall be elected or appointed annually, or at such times as shall be determined by the town councils, for the purposes of this Ordinance, the following officers, who shall receive such compensation, and perform such specific duties as shall from time to time be determined; that is to say:

(1.) A Registrar, who shall be a Doctor of Medicine, whose duty it shall be to record the births, deaths, and marriages, and to regulate all funerals, and the proceedings thereunto appurtenant.

(2.) A Medical Health Officer—who shall be the principal physician-in-ordinary to the Board of Health—who shall superintend, under the direction of the Board of Health, all the sanitary measures ordered by the Board; and who shall advise them generally as to all matter relating to the public health.

(3.) A Board of Consulting Physicians, who shall be elected annually, and whose duty it shall be, in case of an alarm of any contagious or other dangerous disease occurring in the district, to give the Board of Health all such professional advice and information as they may request, with a view to the prevention of such disease, and at all convenient times, when requested, to aid and assist them with their counsel and advice in all matters that relate to the preservation of the health of the inhabitants.

(4.) An Engineer, or Surveyor, whose duty it shall be to furnish all plans required for the use of the Board; to advise in relation to the construction and grade of the streets; the structure of the drains; the water-supply; and, generally, with regard to all plans for improving the surface and substratum of the district.

(5.) Superintendents of Streets, of Health (or Cleaning), of Drains, and of Burials; whose duty it shall be to supervise, and direct, and execute the details of the various departments to which they shall be assigned, under the direction of the Board, of the Health Officer, or of such other persons as the Board of Health may direct.

(6.) Such other officers as the councils may from time to time determine.

LX. Any person who shall violate the provisions of this Ordinance, or any of them; or who shall obstruct the Board, or any of its authorized agents, in the performance of their lawful duties; or who shall do any act or acts by which the public health is endangered—shall be fined therefor not less than dollars, nor more than dollars, for each and every offense, and he shall be subjected to such other penalty as the Board of Health, with the approval of the councils, may fix and determine, and which are not repugnant to the Constitution and laws of the State, or in violation of the regulations of the General Board of Health.

LXI. If any person feel aggrieved by any order of the Board of Health, or by the orders or acts of any of its accredited officers or agents, he shall always have the right of appeal to the Board of Health; or, if he so elect, he may prosecute such appeal in the courts of law, in accordance with the Bill of Rights, as in such cases made and provided; but no such appeal shall be entertained by the Board of Health, unless said appeal is made within four months next after making such order, or the doing of such act, nor unless ten days' notice, in writing, is given to the party against whom the appeal is brought, stating the nature and grounds thereof; nor then, unless the appellant enter into sureties duly to abide the decision of the Board, or to prosecute his appeal in the proper Court.

LXII. All Ordinances and parts of Ordinances heretofore passed, inconsistent with this Ordinance, are hereby repealed.

APPENDIX A.

FORM OF RETURN.

The Health Officer, or Inspector, after ascertaining the condition of his district, shall make his report in the following manner, viz.:

"Health Officer, A. B. , District , reports the condition of premises No. , street, to be as follows:

1. PREVALENT SICKNESS.
   (Under this head state what the disease is, and how many are affected.)
2. OVERCROWDING.
   (State in figures the number of persons occupying the the rooms or houses in *badly situated localities.*)
3. VENTILATION.
   (State if there is any; and, if so, whether it is by doors, windows, or fire-places; especially *when the apartments are closed at night.*)
4. DRAINAGE.
   (State simply if there is *any,* and whether it is "*good*" or "*bad.*"
5. FILTH AND RUBBISH.
   (State the kind, quantity (by estimate), and its specific locality.)
6. WATER SUPPLY.
   (State if there is a supply of water for *cooking, washing,* or *bathing,* and of *what kind.*)
7. DEAD BODIES IN SINGLE LIVING ROOMS.
   (State the cause of death, and the general condition of the apartment and its inhabitants.)

He shall also make a record, in a book to be furnished him for that purpose, of the same facts in tabular form.

APPENDIX B.

FORM OF NOTICE TO ABATE NUISANCES.

(To be served by any Officer competent to serve a civil process.)

CITY OF

OFFICE OF BOARD OF HEALTH, 18

To *No.* *St.*

SIR:—Your premises having been examined, and ascertained to be in a condition which is, in my opinion, prejudicial to the public health, by reason of
you are hereby required, in conformity with the provisions of an Order of the Board of Health, passed to
within hours.

Health Officer.

Approved.

Chairman Committee of Board of Health.

EXTRACT FROM THE ORDER.

"*Ordered,* That the Medical Health Officer, with the concurrence of the Committee of the Board, be and he is hereby authorized to take such measures in regard to causes or occasions of danger to the public health of the city, as he may deem necessary and proper for its preservation."

REPORT

UPON

SEWERAGE, WATER SUPPLY, AND OFFAL.

By JOHN H. GRISCOM, M.D., of New York.

REPORT.

In his artificial condition of civilization, there are two classes of circumstances which effect the health of man: 1st, Those which are found exclusively *within* his domocile; and 2d, Those which are more particularly operative *without* his dwelling. To the former class belong the various impurities of the atmosphere derived from respiration, combustion, and exuberant moisture, the quality of food, the clothing, and personal cleanliness. Included in the latter, or extra-domiciliary causes of disease are terrestrial emanations, meteoric changes, and the influence of those matters, which, having been cast out from the dwelling, are suffered to undergo decomposition in its vicinity.

To me has been assigned the duty of reporting upon "the importance of an ample supply of water, an edequate sewerage, and the proper disposal of offal."

The first of these objects of inquiry—water—belongs to both classes of circumstances, *i. e.*, the internal and external domiciliary. Used as a beverage, for cooking, for bathing, for washing, and cleansing generally, it pertains to the internal affairs of the household; as a means of cooling the atmosphere, of absorbing free gases, of cleansing the ways, and of removing filth, its applications are chiefly external, and in this direction, though more extensive as regards area, they are less important than in their indoor relations.

Of the vast importance of an ample supply of water for family use, an impression may perhaps be best formed by imagining the horrors of a drought, in contrast with the comforts of an abundance of this element furnished unstintedly; and the measure of the comfort and health of a people, or even of a single household, may be judged by the approach to one or the other of these extremes, of the water afforded to, and used by them. There is nothing extravagant in the conjecture, that, in many of the very crowded portions of cities, where dwellings rise to the height of five or six stories, up to which it is impossible, by hand labor, to carry an ample supply of water, that there, suffering and sickness from the deficiency, are marked and decided, while nearer the ground, the inhabitants, being better able to observe rules of cleanliness, and to use it more freely in every way, are on this account less prone to evils of many kinds.

Water should be second only to air in abundance and accessibility; as the poorest has no excuse for self-privation of air, nature pressing it upon him with the force of fifteen pounds to the square inch, and he having only to expand his chest to receive it, so should water be accessible to every one, the poorest more especially, simply by the opening of a valve, that there might be no excuse for its neglect. Stephen Girard and John Jacob Astor could have made no better disposition of their wealth, than to have given the waters of the Schuylkill and the Croton to their fellow-citizens without price.

Passing to the subject of sewerage, we have to observe that terrene exhalations in rural localities are a well-known cause of various diseases, which need not be here enumerated. From this cause every city should and can be, made almost wholly free. However vicious may be the soil upon which a city stands, a thorough system of paving and sewerage will prevent the natural exhalations, and obviate the diseases which will otherwise flow from them. But however well paved and sewered a city may be, whereby its natural exhalations are obviated, the formation of *artificial* marshes above the stones of the pavement, and beyond the reach of the sewers, by the accumulation of the offal of men and animals is equally bad, if not worse. The marsh miasm of new countries which produces intermittent, remittent, and bilious fevers, the scourges of uncultivated regions, is the result of *vegetable* decomposition only ; but if to this there be added a large proportion of animal matter, and the exhalations of the combined decomposition are suffered to invade our dwellings and surround us continually, the intensity of the malarious poison is redoubled, and in addition to the diseases just mentioned, we have Diarrhœa, Dysentery, Cholera, Typhus Fever, and a general depression of the vital powers, which renders every other disorder more dangerous. Of such a character is the miasm of a city of uncleaned and unwashed streets, where the *debris* of the kitchens and manufactories are allowed to accumulate on the surface, exposed to the decomposing influences of the air, the sun, and the rains, and where the fecal emanations of the inhabitants are *preserved* in sinks and cess-pools.

If even the tidal waters of such a magnificent sewer as the river Thames are insufficient to relieve the city of London of the pernicious effects of its vast amount of animal and vegetable *debris* and exhalation, how clean soever its surface may be kept, how much more offensive and deleterious must be the compound animal and vegetable malaria from these same materials, stagnant upon the surface. They form artificial marshes more dangerous than the Pontine.

" The sewerage of large towns and cities consists of refuse animal matters, of the excrementitial discharges of the inhabitants and myriads of the lower animals, of the blood and animal fluids from slaughter-houses, knackers' yards, and tan-pits, of the foul and contaminated waters from gas-works, factories, and other establishments, and of refuse vegetable matters in a state of decomposition from public markets and other places."* The combined amount of these matters is estimated at seven cubic feet (about fifty gallons) per diem, for each individual, which for the city of New York, with a population of 700,000, rises to the daily average of 35,000,000 gallons, and, annually, to the astounding quantity of twelve billions seven hundred and seventy-five millions of gallons (12,775,000,000).

To descant upon the necessity of the immediate and thorough removal of this prodigious mass of waste animal, vegetable, mineral, and gaseous matter, which, were it possible to concentrate it daily, in separate deposits, would require for each day, a reservoir fifty per cent. larger than the Croton distributing reservoir on Murray Hill, New York City; to descant upon the absolute necessity of an immediate removal of these immense masses of poisonous matter far away from the precincts of human lungs; to discuss the fearful results which would follow their retention—would seem to be a work of supererogation; and yet we find even intelligent citizens and legislators, almost everywhere, doubting, hesitating, and procrastinating.

To all such we commend earnestly, and in the pure spirit of patriotism, the following passages from the recent able work on Hygiene, before quoted. The remarks there made, though written for the metropolis of Great Britain, are equally applicable to New York, Philadelphia, or any other large and crowded city.

"In all large cities and towns there are plague-spots where fever of the intermittent, remittent, or continued form always prevails in greater or less intensity. There are districts and localties in our modern Babylon which are ever remitting the poison which generates Typhus Fever; there

* Hygiene, by Dr. Pickford.

are certain squares and streets, nay, particular houses, the inmates of which, family after family, for a long series of years have been the victims of Typhus Fever, though the districts in which they are situated are airy, and the soil dry.

"Open and imperfect sewers, faulty, superficial, choked up and overflowing drains, imperfect traps of cess-pools and water-closets, a filthy condition of the earth's surface, together with intramural burying-grounds, slaughter-houses, and slaughtering-cellars, and the conversion of tidal rivers into cloacæ maximæ, are the fruitful sources of fevers, diarrhœa, and dysentery, in all congregations, and on any one spot, of great multitudes of human beings.

"There is probably no subject so complex, so incalculably difficult to grapple with, especially if it be how to apply a remedy, as the drainage and sewerage of large overgrown cities. Yet, we must perceive, that unless this be efficiently done, an *ultimate limit is set by the hand of man himself to dynasties, to peoples, and to nations.* The air we breathe, loaded with carbonaceous matter, sulphurous and sulphuric acid, sulphate of ammonia, and sulphurretted hydrogen, is deprived, by the absence of vegetation, of the revivifying principle, oxygen, and is hence less fitted for the necessary changes of the blood effected during respiration. The earth which we tread under our feet, loaded with the ashes of our forefathers, and rich with the remains of animal and vegetable matter of ages long gone by, saturated with the putrefying contents of myriads of cess-pools and leaking sewers of our own day, emits at certain seasons of the year the poisonous emanations which generate Typhus, Diarrhœa, Dysentery, and Cholera; whilst the waters of our principal tidal rivers, converted into open common sewers, teem with pestiferous exhala-

16

tions, charged with the germ of disease, or the messenger of death, If, under these favoring conditions, a pestilential epidemic invade our shores, it finds us an unprepared and easy prey.

"The government of every state and nation would do wisely to appoint a minister of public health, whose duty it should be to superintend and watch over the health of the community at large, to see that due ventilation is observed in all large and public buildings, and in the dwellings of the poor; to ascertain that the water is pure, and its supply ample; to prevent all noxious and unwholesome trades and manufactures being carried on within a given distance from towns and dwellings; to prohibit intramural burial-grounds, slaughter-houses, and slaughtering-cellars; but, above all, to lay down, and carry out an effectual, efficient, complete, and common-sense plan of drainage and sewerage for every town and city.

"Were the fearful consequences which result from the reprehensible practice of converting our rivers into open common sewers but thoroughly understood, and properly understood, and properly estimated by the public, no expenditure of time or money would be deemed too great to put an end, by penal enactment, to a system so disgusting, so revolting, and so destructive to the health and lives of the community at large; but more especially of those whose avocations necessitate their daily and hourly exposure to, and residence in the midst of its pernicious influence.

"Unless this montrous and suicidal evil be staid, London will ultimately become the hot-bed of plague and pestilence, and will, as a consequence, be depopulated and deserted, and numbered with the cities of the world which have been. Then, perhaps, may be fulfilled the prophetic visions of Volney, of Walpole, of Shelley, of Macaulay: 'when London shall be an habitation of bitterns; when St. Paul's and Westminster

Abbey shall stand shapeless and nameless ruins, *in the midst of an unpeopled marsh;* when the piers of Westminster Bridge shall become the nuclei of islets of reeds and osiers, and cast the shadows of their broken arches on the solitary stream;' or with Macaulay: 'when travelers from distant regions shall in vain labor to decipher on some mouldering pedestal the name of our proudest chief; shall hear savage hymns chanted to some misshapen idol over the ruined dome of our proudest temple, and shall see a single naked fisherman wash his nets in the river of the ten thousand masts.' "

www.ingramcontent.com/pod-product-compliance
Lightning Source LLC
LaVergne TN
LVHW020312110826
845148LV00017BA/353
* 9 7 8 1 4 2 5 5 2 1 4 3 1 *